the Truth about FIBER in your food

Books by Lawrence Galton

The Disguised Disease: Anemia
Don't Give Up on an Aging Parent
The Silent Disease: Hypertension
Freedom from Backaches
Your Inner Conflicts
How Long Will You Live?
The Laboratory of the Body
The Family Book of Preventive Medicine
with Benjamin F. Miller, M.D.
Freedom from Heart Attacks
with Benjamin F. Miller, M.D.
Your Heart: Complete Information for the Family
with William Likoff, M.D., and Bernard Segal, M.D.
Adult Physical Fitness Manual, President's Council on Physical Fitness

the Truth about FIBER in your food

LAWRENCE GALTON

Introduction by
Denis P. Burkitt, M.D., F.R.S., F.R.C.S.

CROWN PUBLISHERS, INC., NEW YORK

 Inquiries should be addressed to Crown Publishers, Inc., One Park Avenue, New York, N.Y. 10016.
Printed in the United States of America
Published simultaneously in Canada by General Publishing Company Limited

Library of Congress Cataloging in Publication Data

Galton, Lawrence.
The truth about fiber in your food.

Includes bibliographical references and index.
1. Fiber deficiency diseases. 2. High-fiber diet.
I. Title.
RC627.F5G34 613.2′6 75-34144
ISBN 0-517-52504-6

Second Printing, March, 1976

dedicated with esteem
and affection to my
editors, Paul Nadan and
Herbert Michelman, who
did so much to encourage
and help in the
research for and writing
of this book

Contents

Introduction

An impressive array of evidence has been brought to light and pieced together by many workers to show the great importance to health of a hitherto neglected component of human food, the unabsorbable fiber, or roughage.

This important knowledge can be put to maximum practical use only if it is presented to the lay public in a form that can be easily understood, and in an accurate and balanced manner.

This is what Lawrence Galton, an experienced and competent medical journalist, has both attempted and achieved.

He has rightly emphasized that present knowledge of the potentially harmful results of refining carbohydrate foods is the result of the efforts of many researchers in different countries making complementary observations. Their individual contributions may be likened to the various and widely differing components of the human body, each providing its different but distinctive and often indispensable contribution to the working of the whole.

If any one individual were to be singled out for special mention it might be Surgeon Captain T. L. Cleave, R.N., who was probably the first to cogently argue that a number of apparently unconnected diseases characteristic of modern Western civilization might in fact be merely differing results of a common causative factor.

With a discovery of this nature there is always the danger of those with a superficial grasp of the argument both overstating the case and failing to make the all important differentiation between fact and hypothesis. Although a few of the diseases discussed in this book fall into the former category, the majority must still be considered to lie in the latter. Another error has been on the overemphasis of the value of adding fiber to a fiber-depleted diet, without realizing that this is merely a compromise. This will probably benefit or confer some protection against the intestinal diseases referred to, and those postulated to relate to the straining required to evacuate unnaturally hard stools.

Present knowledge, however, suggests that starch and sugar must be eaten within the fibrous cell wall within which they are found in nature to prevent some of the diseases listed. It is important to underline these facts and Mr. Galton has been careful to do so. There is already available a multitude of synthetic bulk-forming products offered as substitutes for a change to fiber-rich foods, but any of these must be considered a second best.

Mr. Galton's book reads like an exciting detective novel, and such it is, but its potential value is vastly greater than the mere interest of the story. If his advice is heeded, the amount of suffering that could be prevented is great indeed, and the real reward of any true medical scientist must surely be the knowledge that his efforts have benefited many, rather than the recognition that is accorded to his work.

–Denis P. Burkitt, M.D., F.R.S., F.R.C.S.
member British Medical Research Council
and co-discoverer of the importance of
fiber in the diet

1

Overview

EVERY once in a while something of extraordinary importance occurs in the scientific world—extraordinary because it unmistakably touches the lives of all of us.

This book is the story of such an event and of the scientific search that led to it.

It now appears that with our modern technology we have once again outsmarted ourselves. By refining out of our diet an essential ingredient, dietary fiber—although it was not known to be essential before, and even the name is new—we have opened the way for a remarkable variety of diseases, some of them chronic, nagging nuisances even if not critical to life, others deadly, and all of them previously puzzling in many ways.

At first blush it is bound to seem incredible that any single factor, especially a long-dismissed dietary one, could play any role in such seemingly disparate diseases as these: in the gut—appendicitis, diverticular disease (abnormal outpouchings of the large bowel), polyps of the large bowel, cancer of the bowel, irritable colon, hiatal hernia, gallbladder disease; outside the gut—diabetes, atherosclerosis and coronary artery disease, obesity, hemorrhoids, varicose veins, thrombophlebitis, and dental disease.

Yet, there is impressive evidence now that this single deficiency that affects most if not all of us can account either in part or in whole for these ills. Correction of the deficiency already has produced striking benefits for people with some conditions that respond relatively quickly to correction, and the evidence indicates that correction over a longer period may well produce no less striking benefits in many and perhaps all the remaining conditions.

At this point a pertinent word about that deficiency.

It is, ironically enough, a deficiency of a dietary material long assumed inert, unneeded, undigested, without nutritional or any other value. Sometimes old wives' tales turn out to have some validity. This is one instance—for our grandmothers recognized a few virtues in what they called "roughage," although nutritionists of the time scoffed.

Dietary fiber is more than roughage; in fact, as it turns out, it is not roughage at all.

And, curiously, although it may have no nutritional value and is not even absorbed from the human gut, dietary fiber has much to do with the environment of the gut and, through that, can exert profound influences even outside the gut.

Dietary fiber is *not* merely a matter of bran—although some have hastily leaped to the conclusion that it is and there is some tendency now to regard bran as a new modern panacea. It is no panacea.

Dietary fiber is removed by modern refining processes from many of our most commonly used foods. It is present in other foods, which many of us make little use of or handle in such ways as to seriously impair their fiber value.

Bran, of course, contains fiber. But merely taking several spoonfuls of bran a day is not the answer because the evidence is that fiber in its natural state in foods has—as the result of being actually a part of those foods—effects and values not to be duplicated by bran alone. A concentration on bran alone can be medically irresponsible, according to those pioneering in dietary fiber research, as the evidence here will show.

The story of the discovery of the vital importance of dietary fiber is fascinating—and all the more so because of the men involved.

They range from an Irish surgeon who spent twenty years in Africa and became world-famed for his discovery and cure of a dread cancer of children . . . to a distinguished English physician who established the nature of the disease kwashiorkor, opening the way for its effective treatment . . . to one of the world's renowned medical mathematicians who had much to do with linking lung cancer and smoking . . . to an indomitable surgeon-captain of the British navy who evolved, years ago, a theory of disease that he stuck by even though long ridiculed.

There are many others in what has come to be known as Britain's "Fiber Gang," but which is now rapidly becoming a worldwide fiber gang.

I am greatly indebted to all of them for the generous amount of time they spent with me and the total help they provided for the preparation of this book. I have the feeling that many readers will be no less grateful to them.

What follows is their story, the work they have done and are continuing to do, the evidence they have developed—and you will, I think, be able to judge the quality and significance of that evidence and the worth of acting upon it. Much of what you read throughout you can act upon immediately, but in a final chapter you will find a program of detailed practical suggestions based on the work of these men.

2

Mr. Burkitt returns

IN 1966, when Denis Burkitt came home to England from Africa, he had no idea of what, totally unplanned, lay ahead for him.

He was returning from a remarkable experience that had made him world-famed, and his intention was to devote the rest of his life to carrying further the work he had done in Africa.

Trained as a surgeon, awarded a fellowship at the Royal College of Surgeons in 1938 when he was only twenty-seven, Mr. Burkitt—for so he was entitled to be addressed as surgeons in Britain traditionally are—had been posted by the army during World War II to Africa. After the war, rather than take up a lucrative practice in England that would virtually have been assured by his fellowship, he chose to become a government surgeon in Uganda.

And he was a busy general surgeon for twelve years until one day he was introduced to a dread and puzzling disease of children, fatal within a few weeks to a few months, puzzling because it seemed like a malignancy, but unlike malignancies struck in more than one place at once, sometimes producing large symmetrical swellings on both sides of the upper and lower jaws.

It was to become known as Burkitt's lymphoma. In years of patient work Burkitt established that it was a malignancy and that it not only struck in the jaws but could take other forms, manifesting itself without involving the jaws, becoming apparent as an abdominal, kidney, or other tumor.

And yet, although it proved to be, in its various forms, the most common tumor in African children (and was later found in the United States and Europe as well), Burkitt soon found that it did not occur all over Africa.

On a 10,000-mile safari through twelve African countries in an old Ford station wagon accompanied by two missionary friends, Burkitt pinpointed where it occurred and where it did not. He found rainfall and temperature to be critical factors, the lymphoma occurring where rainfall exceeded 30 inches annually and temperature never fell below 60° F.

It was remarkable epidemiologic work done on a pittance. It pointed to a virus as cause. Then, refusing to give up on treatment, which previously had been useless, Burkitt began experimenting with drugs—first vincristine, then cyclophosphamide. By 1966, when he left Africa, he was getting total clinical remissions and long-term survival in more than 40 percent of cases, and this would be improved by others who took over his therapeutic work.*

When he came home to England it was to join the staff of the British Medical Research Council in London. Here he had support for broadening his work. Because plotting the geography of Burkitt's lymphoma had been so productive, he wanted to turn to studies of the geography of a number of other tumors, among them cancer of the stomach, cancer of the esophagus, cancer of the penis, Kaposi's sarcoma, which occurs almost exclusively in Africa, and other lymphomas.

He did turn to them—and then came the telephone call about a year after he had returned home.

There was a touch of irony in it. It was to make him realize

---

* Among the many honors bestowed on Denis Burkitt is the 1972 Lasker Award, one of American medicine's highest distinctions, the citation for which read:

"In 1956, Mr. Burkitt, working in East Africa, was first to recognize that tumors appearing in characteristic sites and often occurring in the same individuals, were really different manifestations of the same type of tumor.

"The surgical treatment of the disease was highly unsatisfactory and no radiotherapy was available in East Africa. His early treatment in 1961 with chemotherapy was remarkably successful and led to the elaboration of a number of chemotherapeutic programs for the treatment of the disease.

"It was his recognition and clear description of this tumor which led to its use as a model for the development of other chemotherapeutic regimens and the extrapolation of information gained in those studies to other kinds of cancer.

"Mr. Burkitt's work also brought a stimulus to leukemia chemotherapy and to studies of host defense mechanisms in cancer, and to the possible causation of human cancer by viruses."

that something perhaps even more significant than the epidemiological cues for Burkitt's lymphoma had been there, virtually under his nose, all the time he had worked in Africa and he had not realized it. It was to change the course of his life and work.

The telephone call came from Sir Richard Doll, M.D., medical statistician, regius professor of medicine at Oxford, one of the world's distinguished medical scientists, and a colleague of Burkitt on the Medical Research Council.

"Denis," said Sir Richard, "I'd like you to meet a chap named Cleave. He is most interesting, and I think his work and ideas would interest you. There is much in what he says which, as a statistician, I could easily poke holes in. But I have a hunch he may be right nevertheless."

Burkitt saw Cleave—Surgeon-Captain T. L. Cleave—Peter to his friends. He was to see him many times.

3

The meeting

CLEAVE'S ideas were, indeed, interesting. They were, in fact, eye-poppingly astonishing. Burkitt listened.

Cleave's thesis was nothing less than that man, by trying to outwit nature, had let himself in for multiple grief, and did not realize what he had done—including the introduction of a host of pressing diseases. And yet, if only he did and made amends, he could be rid of those diseases.

"You may drive out nature with a pitchfork," Cleave liked to say, quoting Horace, "yet she will ever hurry back, to triumph in stealth over your foolish contempt."

It was Cleave's utter conviction that nature, from a practical point of view, is never wrong as long as she is acting in a natural environment—that is to say, the environment in which the organism concerned has been evolved.

All species, including man, Cleave argued, adapt over time to their environment—and if there is a change in the environment, it will take time for man or any other species to adapt.

But there had occurred with relative suddenness a marked change in the food environment for man. It was man's own doing. It was a more profound change than man had ever imagined. There had been no opportunity—in time—for adaptation to take place.

And the consequences were profound.

They consisted of a series of diseases that had never before been considered as being all consequences of an alteration in food. Yet, to Cleave, they clearly were.

There had been two main ways in which man had altered food from its natural state. The first was by cooking—a common habit so long that there had been enough time for some adaptation to it.

In any case, cooking would not have had serious consequences. Actually, boiling, Cleave noted, may parallel and facilitate the first stages of digestion. Other forms of cooking, particularly overcooking, could somewhat hinder digestion, presenting the gastric juice with coagulated and even charred protein, making it more difficult for the juice to diffuse through and combine with it. And this is even more the case if frying has coated the protein with fat, which is relatively resistant to digestive activity in the stomach. One consequence could be less neutralizing power of the food on the gastric juice and encouragement of peptic ulcer formation.

But it was the second alteration in food—concentration by machinery—that was by far the more serious.

"Concentration," Cleave declared, "affects, for practical purposes, only one class of food—the carbohydrates. Whole-meal flour is turned into white flour, and the bran rejected; the pulp of the sugarcane and the sugar beet have the sugar extracted in almost pure form, and the balance of the pulp is then likewise rejected. Now whereas cooking has been going on in the human race for probably 200,000 years, so many thousands of years in fact that our jaws show at least some evolutionary adaptation to it, just as the loss of body hair shows an adaptation to the wearing of clothes, there is no question yet of our being adapted to the concentration of carbohydrates by machinery. Such processes have been in existence little more than a century for the ordinary man and from an evolutionary point of view this counts as nothing at all."

Many of our ills today, Cleave was convinced, are an expression of the one fact—that we are not yet adapted to the concentration of carbohydrates by machinery.

And among the ills he named were constipation, diverticular disease, irritable colon, and cancer of the colon; varicose veins, deep venous thrombosis, and hemorrhoids; dental disease and peptic ulcer; obesity, diabetes, and coronary disease.

These, in fact, Cleave argued, could be looked upon not so much as separate diseases but really as all varying manifestations of a single disease, which he called the Saccharine Disease. "Saccharine," Cleave emphasized, should be pronounced like the river Rhine to sharply differentiate it from the chemical sweetener saccharine (which is pronounced reen in England), and means "related to sugar."

The many manifestations of the saccharine disease had become rampant in developed nations, Cleave argued, due in part to the lack of fiber removed by modern machinery and to a greater extent to the overconsumption of sugar made possible, convenient, tasty, and tempting by machine concentration—both sugar as sugar and sugar into which refined starches are quickly converted in the body.

They were not rampant in the underdeveloped nations, he argued. They were rare in rural Africa. When they began to increase in the underdeveloped countries, it was not in the rural areas where people retained their tribal diets but in the cities among people adopting Western customs and diet.

Cleave argued thus for years before he met Denis Burkitt. In 1956 he wrote a medical paper entitled "The Neglect of Natural Principles in Current Medical Practice." It was published in of all places the *Journal of the Royal Naval Medical Service*. No attention.

He wrote several books and many letters to British medical journals. They attracted little attention, and often when his arguments were noted at all they were ridiculed.

Burkitt did not ridicule them.

As he listened to Cleave, he suddenly realized that all the time he had been in Africa he had had an impression that the diseases Cleave spoke of as being rare there were, indeed, apparently rare but he had given no thought as to why.

Nor, from his experience with Burkitt's lymphoma, was he inclined to dismiss out of hand the idea that many seemingly disparate diseases could be manifestations of one underlying disease or at least related to a single cause.

Burkitt was to listen repeatedly to Cleave, hearing the whole story of how he had come to his radical concept.

4

The "bran man" who wasn't

PETER Cleave is sixty-nine and officially retired from the navy. "But," he says, "while it is definitely true that I am long in the tooth, it is a bloody lie that I am retired; I work harder now at medicine than ever in my life."

He began working at medicine very young. He was twenty-one when, after training at St. Mary's Hospital in London and the Royal Infirmary in Bristol, he entered the navy as a doctor.

For the first half of his career in the navy he served aboard ship and in naval hospitals. During the last half he was director of medical research at the Institute of Naval Medicine.

It was during his service in World War II aboard the battleship *King George V*—noted among other things for its chase of the German battleship *Bismarck*—that Cleave had some large-scale practical experiences that very much influenced his thinking.

There were 1,500 men aboard and while they were not constipated down to the last man, he recalls, most were because of the difficulty in getting fresh vegetables and fresh fruit aboard ship in wartime.

"We had many tinned vegetables aboard—tinned turnips, tinned carrots, tinned everything. On one occasion I received a rebuke from the captain of the ship, a great friend of mine, when, at Scapa Flow, I saw sheep eating raw natural turnips, couldn't help thinking how much better off we would be on board if we had those turnips rather than the cooked analogs, and asked permission to land several thousand tins of our turnips for the sheep ashore while we took on board their raw manglewoozies for ourselves."

Cleave himself was no exception to the general rule of constipation on board. And he decided to try an experiment in treating himself. Bran is the fiber-rich, outer husk of any grain. It is bran that is discarded in the milling of white flour. Some of it is processed into special bran cereal preparations. Much of it is fed to animals. Unprocessed bran at the mill is far cheaper than the processed preparations that in fact have long been used by some of the constipated (although relatively very few in comparison with the numbers using laxatives or, as they are called in England, aperients). Cleave tried the unprocessed bran on himself, not only because it was cheaper but also because he had a feeling for using natural things rather than processed whenever he could.

Cleave became a popular man aboard the *King George V*. After experimenting with double satisfaction on himself—satisfaction over the elimination of his constipation and over the ability of natural raw bran to do it—he began to parcel it out to all victims of constipation.

"We dispensed it," he recalls, "by the hundredweight." This, so far as he can tell, was the first time the raw bran had been used for the purpose.

Hemorrhoids constituted another naval curse. It seemed to Cleave that constipation was the basic reason for these "piles," which, much like varicose veins in the legs, are unnaturally dilated blood vessels. As he saw it, in a constipated person, with the rectum full of hardened feces that have no right to be there, the fecal masses exert pressure on veins in the rectal wall—and, largely comparable to what happens when you produce pressure by circling one wrist with the other hand and squeezing so the veins stand out—the rectal wall veins balloon.

Cleave found that bran, while it did not remove any large, long-standing hemorrhoidal masses, did provide gratifying relief for the vast numbers of hemorrhoid-troubled aboard.

In 1946 Cleave was serving at the Royal Naval Hospital in Chatham where, as he puts it, he "had the good fortune" of working with another surgeon-commander who was suffering from diverticular disease. The disorder involves the formation of little outpouchings of the large intestine, which may trap intestinal contents and become inflamed. It is, today, a very common disorder.

Cleave's colleague agreed to his suggestion to try bran. "He achieved salvation with it," Cleave says. Shortly, all patients turning up at the hospital with diverticular disease were being placed on bran.

It was hardly any wonder that Peter Cleave became known in the British navy as the great "bran man." And he was sometimes the object of ridicule as word got around that with Cleave bran was a panacea and that he was also inordinately fond of bananas.

Cleave's wife, Helen, recalls that even many years later she would repeatedly meet old acquaintances at the naval club and at parties who would greet her: "Hello, Helen, are you still living on bran and bananas?"

"Sometimes," Helen Cleave says, "I used to feel quite huffy and would say, 'Well, we have very nice food; come to lunch or dinner, and you'll have something more than bran and bananas.'"

Bran hardly constituted a panacea for Cleave.

His thinking went far beyond. He was to consider the many possible consequences of the removal of fiber from the modern diet not only in terms of the loss of the fiber itself but also in terms of overconsumption promoted by fiberless foods. Bran might compensate to some extent for the fiber removal. Overconsumption was another matter—and, in Cleave's thinking, a vital one, productive of a whole series of diseases of its own.

Long before Cleave, some attention had been paid to what seemed to be direct consequences of fiber removal through the refining of cereals.

Flour, of course, had been refined from cereal grains for millennia. Generally, the refining—the removal of the outer coat or husk of the kernels—had been light. But even among the ancient Egyptians there were efforts to obtain a highly refined white flour that would offer a more luxurious taste than coarse whole flour when used for bread or cake. In a process called bolting, the flour was filtered through a cloth sieve. Such flour, being expensive, went only to the wealthy while the poor ate coarse grain.

About 1870 the roller mill was developed, and the separation of the bran, germ, and white inner substance of grain became far more rapid and inexpensive. Not until fifty years later was there any realization that most of the grain's vitamins and minerals are concentrated in the bran and germ that had been considered useless and had been fed largely to animals. It was hardly likely that the full values of bran and germ, beyond their vitamin and mineral content, were known, although the usefulness of unbolted flour as a laxative *had* been known ever since the time of Hippocrates, father of medicine, 400 years before Christ.

In America early in the nineteenth century, Sylvester Graham, for whom graham flour and graham crackers were named, extolled the importance of not discarding any part of the grain. Among other things, he pointed to the fact that livestock could not be healthy without bulk along with grain and suggested that whole grains could relieve many cases of human constipation—and, yes, even diarrhea.

During the Revolutionary War, Baron von Steuben, a German officer who trained American soldiers, often observed that Prussian soldiers were notably healthy and, in his opinion, this was due to the use of unbolted bread.

In the late eighteenth century, during the war with France, 80,000 English soldiers in Essex had to eat bread made from unbolted flour after Parliament enacted a law designed to stretch the supply of grain. At first, the soldiers cordially detested it but within a few weeks came to prefer it, and the improvement in their health apparently was great enough so that whole-grain bread became widely popular in England. But when the law expired and refined flour became available again from the United States, white bread gradually came back into use.

Similarly, in England during both world wars, coarse flour was used in order to stretch the supply of grain and a general improvement in health was noted. But, after each war, there was a return to white flour because, it was said, the white spoiled less easily, was needed by bakers to make more appealing products, and farmers needed the bran and germ for their livestock, and anyhow other foods could supply the known nutrients lost in the refining of flour.

There had also been the experience in Denmark in 1917 when a severe drought, coupled with the Allied blockade, threatened starvation. At that point 80 percent of the pigs and two-thirds of the cattle in Denmark were ordered slaughtered so the cereals thus saved could be fed to the population in the form of whole rye bread to which was added 12 to 15 percent of wheat bran.

The reported results were dramatic. In the first year after introduction of the new bread, mortality from all causes in Denmark declined by 17 percent to the lowest level ever noted in any country up to then. During the 1918 worldwide influenza pandemic, Denmark was the only country experiencing no increase in the death rate; in fact, the Danish mortality rate from all causes actually decreased while the rate in other countries in Europe increased by as much as 46 percent.

Perhaps the most eminent proponent of whole grains was a renowned English surgeon, Sir Arbuthnot Lane, who, in a book entitled *The Prevention of Diseases Peculiar to Civilization,* wrote that "the greatest of all physicians, Hippocrates, used to urge upon the citizens of Athens that it was essential that they should pass large bulky motions after every meal, and that to ensure this they had to eat abundantly of whole-meal bread, vegetables and fruits. . . . On this I can only comment that the modern doctor is not following the precepts and practice of his great predecessor, and that knowledge of diet has not formed an integral part of his education."

To Cleave it began to seem that just one result of removal of fiber from the diet was this simple, direct chain of events: without the bulk provided by fiber, the passage of intestinal contents was impeded, and so—constipation. Diverticular disease was a complication of the constipation. And the pressure of constipated masses in the colon on the great venous trunks coming up from the legs was decisive in the production of varicose veins and, much more important, dreaded deep vein thrombosis that may make a nightmare of any surgical operation as it leads to a clot in a leg vein that may break off, travel upward to a lung, producing life-threatening pulmonary embolism.

Cleave began to see another group of diseases, major diseases—most notably diabetes, obesity, and coronary thrombosis—as being due not to lack of fiber itself but to overconsumption engendered by the removal of fiber.

Refined sugar, he became convinced, was the major culprit. It is even more refined than white flour. Between 1815 and the present sugar intake in England increased from about 15 pounds per person per year to about 120 pounds—and much the same thing happened in the United States and other Western countries.

To be sure, Cleave acknowledged, man had always had a taste for sugar. But the sugar had been found in natural form in fruits.

"Let us suppose," Cleave would say, "that you take sugar in its natural form which, in England, would be the ordinary apple, the quintessence of an English fruit. You would need to eat twenty apples a day to get the amount of sugar we get per day in combinations of foods containing refined table sugar. Or you could eat a three-pound sugar beet to get that amount of sugar, but the beet would be about the size of a child's head. Either way, eating the twenty apples or the sugar beet would be difficult if not impossible, and if by chance you did manage it, you would be eating very little else. But you can lower the equivalent in refined sugar—in cups of tea and the like—easily, without noticing it."

Such overconsumption of refined sugar, Cleave came to think, must have profound consequences. And refined flour contributed because with its digestion in the body it rapidly was converted into sugar.

What would be the consequences? An obvious one, Cleave considered, is obesity. But go beyond that. "Obesity," he would argue, "is associated dramatically with the incidence of diabetes. And also let me add to diabetes—coronary thrombosis. The sequence is very often obesity, high blood sugar, coronary disease. You can get the coronary disease without the intervention of diabetes, but more than half of all diabetics die of coronary disease."

Cleave had been closely in touch with Dr. G. D. Campbell whose work with Natal Indians in South Africa had pointed to the relationship between sugar consumption and both diabetes and coronary heart disease.

Campbell had remarked on the far higher incidence of diabetes in the Natal Indians, heavy sugar users, as compared with the low incidence among Indians in India whose sugar consumption was low. Campbell had formulated a "rule of twenty years"—it took twenty years of sugar consumption to produce overt diabetes. Campbell also reported that Natal Indians, besides being riddled with diabetes, were riddled with coronary heart disease as well.

Another consequence of overconsumption of refined foods and of refined sugar in particular, Cleave came to believe, was a change in the normal microbial flora—the colonies of bacteria—in the large bowel. And it was this change, he argued, that played the dominant role in appendicitis and in infections of the urinary tract, and an important role in gallstones and gallbladder disease.

Nor was Cleave prepared to stop there.

Modern refining methods not only removed fiber; they also removed protein. And it was the loss of protein, he argued, that was responsible for peptic ulcers.

Both gastric and duodenal ulcers, he was convinced, are confined to the eaters of refined carbohydrates and are unknown in those who do not consume these foods. "If anyone will tell me," he says, "that the eaters of this or that unrefined grain do get ulcers, I will tell them, 'Go examine their larders and see if the sugar and white flour and white rice haven't already arrived.' Because I do not believe for one moment that these diseases ever occur under natural circumstances."

Cleave points to the experience of the English and Americans held by the Japanese as prisoners of war. His brother, Surgeon-

Captain H. L. Cleave, was also a prisoner and was in surgical charge of most of the prisoners, both in Tokyo and Hong Kong. The prisoners were nearly all fed on red unmilled rice. There was a dramatic decline in the incidence of both gastric and duodenal ulcers among them.

When grains are refined and the bran removed, much of the protein is also removed because the protein is largely in the bran. In the refining of sugar all the protein is removed.

Why should this encourage ulcers? Cleave argues that, although ulcers have been blamed on either an excess of stomach acid or a failure of the mucin, a mixture of proteins, in the stomach lining to protect against the acid, a third factor is far more important than these two. The protein component in natural food neutralizes the acid, and if the protein is removed in whole or in part the tendency to peptic ulceration increases markedly because the acid is let loose on the mucosal membranes of the stomach.

"Now this neutralization is far more important than hyperacidity or deficient mucin production and I will tell you why," says Cleave. "It is because it is a governable factor. We can govern the neutralization of our acid by taking unrefined food but we cannot govern our acid production or mucin protection. We can make a decisive contribution with food."

Cleave's ideas, even if they were not to be accepted in full, should have triggered interest in all the years he had been trying to be heard. But they didn't; for all intents and purposes, he was in limbo.

A concept of a single causative factor operating in many varied diseases, diseases not commonly considered to have anything to do with each other—a hypothesis that these seemingly distinct and separate diseases are really the same disease manifesting itself in many body systems—was difficult to accept.

Cleave could use analogy. He could point to arsenic poisoning and the established fact that it does not express itself in any one system of the body. It affects the cutaneous system and leads to darkening of the skin. It affects the central nervous system and produces paralysis. It affects the blood, the muscles, breathing. In fact, medical books commonly tabulate the many systems affected by arsenic poisoning.

If you were to take any one manifestation of arsenic poisoning and call it a disease, Cleave could remark, you would end up with many diseases due to arsenic. But arsenic poisoning is really a single disease manifesting itself in more than one system.

So, too, with refined carbohydrates. In the stomach they cause peptic ulcer. When they get into the small intestine and are absorbed in gross excess, they cause overweight, diabetes, and coronary disease. On down in the large bowel, they cause diverticular disease, constipation and, through pressure on veins, varicosities and hemorrhoids. These are not all separate diseases but one disease operating in many bodily systems.

"It would indeed be a remarkable coincidence," Cleave argued, "if all these separate diseases were due to one cause, refined carbohydrates. But if you make them all one disease operating in many systems, it's all comprehensible, not coincidental."

But it was not comprehensible to medical men generally. It seemed to many that Cleave's notions were pure philosophy arrived at largely through armchair speculation.

Rightly or wrongly, even some of his admirers felt that he was not attracting much scientific attention partly because he tended to try to oversell his ideas, was not as critical of them as he might be, bristled at any criticism from others, and responded to it with broadside blasts—and also because he was putting forward a hypothesis that depended upon statistics and epidemiological observations for support, and he had not collected the sort of data that professional epidemiologists would expect him to collect. His data, it seemed to many, came from hearsay, from reports of friends, from other people's books, some of which were not very reliable.

And yet, as Sir Richard Doll has observed: "When you start looking in detail at what Cleave was saying, a lot of it was actually good common sense. A good deal of his facts were true. So that really his ideas deserved a lot more attention than they got."

Burkitt was the man to give and get it.

5

The network

OF Denis Burkitt and the work he had done on lymphoma, one of his closest friends, Dr. Hugh C. Trowell, who had been an early colleague in Africa and shown him his first case of the disease, has remarked: "I know Denis very well and if somebody had suggested back then, early on, that he would make such a striking series of findings, of such great importance, I would have said, 'Denis, no.' He was too quiet and modest. I would have been wrong. He has gifts that really lead to major accomplishments—humility, dogged perseverance, and the ability to see things fresh."

These gifts were to be put to use again now.

To Burkitt, Cleave's ideas were a fresh breeze. They stimulated him. He was not without reservations about some of them from the beginning.

"But I realized," Burkitt says, "that most of what he said was very valid, was of great importance, although people had been laughing at it. As I did more and more research, there were more and more places where I didn't totally agree with him.

"But I feel now, as I did from the beginning, that a lot of Cleave is genius. What makes him all the more an astonishing man is that, although he never had the opportunity of working in developing countries, he had the capacity to sense the differences in disease patterns there and the fortitude to write so many hundreds of letters to people in those countries and all over the world seeking information on which he built his hypothesis. You know, when you have the opportunity of going around and checking and cross-checking, you often find that people tell you something with the best of intentions but when you cross-check it turns out that they are quite wrong. So it is incredible what Cleave put together from correspondence really."

One of the first things Burkitt did after hearing Cleave out was to sit down and write out a précis of what Cleave had been saying. This he sent to many of his missionary friends in Africa. Did it, he wanted to know, ring true in their experience?

Almost unanimously, they replied that, yes, it did; that although they had not thought very much about it until now, it did seem to be true that the diseases Cleave listed as manifestations of his saccharine disease were uncommon, perhaps even quite rare, among rural Africans, Africans living and eating as they had historically, not yet exposed to a Western diet.

After that, Burkitt set to work to try to check in detail what Cleave had been saying.

He used a technique he had devised for the lymphoma work, ingeniously simple, down-to-earth, practical.

After he had seen his first case of lymphoma—in a five-year-old boy with swellings on both sides of both upper and lower jaws, a complete puzzle to other doctors in Africa, a complete puzzle to him—he had only a few weeks later seen another while happening to glance out of a window of one of the wards of a district hospital fifty miles away that he was visiting.

Both children died and, unable to get them out of mind, Burkitt then studied hospital records, first, of all children treated for jaw tumors but then of all children treated for tumors of any kind. And it turned out that the jaw tumor was a lymphoma—a malignancy affecting the lymphatic system, a body circulatory system for the transparent liquid, lymph, that bathes all tissues—and that it could involve not only the jaws but also eyes, ovaries, kidneys, and other body sites and organs.

It was the most common tumor of childhood in Uganda. And yet, Burkitt soon discovered, common as it was in Uganda, it was unknown 2,000 miles away in South Africa. Why? Where did it stop?

All Burkitt could get in the way of a research grant to try to find out was 15 pounds sterling, about $40. With that he printed 1,200 leaflets illustrated with photographs of children with the lymphoma. Out they went, along with a questionnaire asking, "How long have you worked in your hospital and have you seen this condition?," to as many government and mission physicians throughout Africa as he knew about.

And from the responses indicating not only where the condition had been seen but—just as important and even more important—where it had not been seen, Burkitt got clues, later double-checked with his 10,000-mile personal safari, to the geographical distribution of the malignancy, the temperature and humidity conditions governing that distribution, and the likelihood of virus involvement.*

Burkitt had been grateful for, and impressed by, the responses of the mission physicians. And when, back in England, he set to work to try to determine the geography of other cancers, he conceived of the idea of a network of reporting mission hospitals in Africa and India and began to build it.

It was that network that he built up even further—to more than 150 hospitals—and used to check in detail into facts that might buttress Cleave's ideas.

Monthly, from Burkitt's office, a reporting form went to each hospital. Had there been any cases of heart attack, of diabetes? Had any patients with gallstones, or hemorrhoids, or varicose veins, or peptic ulcer, or other specific diseases been seen? If so, who were the patients, what were their circumstances?

To set up the enlarged network, Burkitt visited the hospitals. He talked to the doctors. There are some large mission hospitals, particularly in India—hospitals with 250 beds, staffed by a number of physicians, including surgeons, obstetricians, and other specialists. But most mission hospitals in Africa have only one or two doctors who do everything.

They are dedicated men; they have to be to spend many years in lonely, isolated, difficult circumstances. They know the language; they know the people. But it was essential for Burkitt to convince them of the importance that their reporting would have—and, in particular, of the importance of looking for things about them, in and out of the hospital, for ailments that did exist but, fully as important and perhaps even more so, for those that did not.

Burkitt recalls being impressed in his early days by a conversation with one of Britain's most distinguished medical researchers, Harold Himsworth, now Sir Harold and director of the British Medical Research Council.

---

* For those who are interested, a brief account of the Burkitt lymphoma work and its present status may be found in the Appendix.

"Denis," Himsworth had remarked at one point, "do you remember the story in Sherlock Holmes when Holmes said to Watson: 'The whole clue, as I see it, to this case lies in the behavior of the dog.' And Watson said: 'But, sir, the dog did nothing at all.' 'That,' said Holmes, 'is the whole point.'

"And it often is in medicine," said Himsworth. "The clue can lie in what is not there rather than what is there."

Burkitt often told that story. He had others to tell.

"In the early stages of my study of lymphoma," he would remark, "a chap came over from West Africa. I showed him cases and I asked, do you see them in West Africa. He said, no. But three weeks later, he wrote to say he had seen his first two cases. He was looking now. You have to look for a thing and not see it and then you have something to say.

"On the other hand," Burkitt continued, "I visited a large hospital in India with an enormous department of radiology. And the head of radiology told me that in sixteen years he had seen only nine cases of diverticular disease. When I asked why he hadn't reported this, he said, 'But I never thought I had anything to report!' Yet it is terribly important that he should report it. We want to know where diverticular disease and appendicitis and varicose veins and coronary heart disease and other diseases don't occur. For one thing, that may lead us to something. For another, unless negatives are reported now, a dozen or a score of years from now we will have no base lines and won't be able to say that we had hardly any of this before and now we have a lot."

Burkitt had a tactic that he used often and it worked because he thoroughly believed in what he said. He uses it to this day.

"I sometimes go to a hospital in Africa," he says, "and I say to a chap, 'Good morning, Smith. Do you know, Smith, you're a world authority.' 'Well,' he says, 'blimey, what am I a world authority on, living way out here?' 'Well,' I say, 'you know there is no one in the world who knows more about the disease pattern of this tribe here than you do.' 'Well,' he says, 'come to think of it, you might be right.'

"And as soon as he realizes he is a world authority, I say, 'Get a notebook and a pencil and do a bit of observation.' He says, 'What will I look for, what will I write about?' I say, 'You write down the things you don't see.'

"And before long he is writing to me that he has been watching people's legs for the last year and has seen only two cases of varicose veins. This is news, something worth publishing."

Burkitt's network grew. The reports began to come in. He could begin to accumulate data that had not been available to Cleave.

He could also begin to get scientific attention for the possibly important, perhaps even overriding, role of dietary changes in fomenting many diseases—attention Cleave had not been able to get and attention that would soon produce a remarkable burst of research by scientists of many disciplines.

The attention came, he insists, simply because he had a "platform"; he had become famed for his lymphoma work.

"I know perfectly well," he says, "that if I hadn't got a platform from the work my colleagues and I did on the lymphomas, I wouldn't be allowed to talk about food. They would say Burkitt is a crank. I was talking at a big meeting in Edinburgh not long ago, the meeting of the Royal Medical Society, and a student said to my wife, not knowing she was my wife, 'That was a good talk that Burkitt gave.' But then he said, 'Of course, nobody but Denis Burkitt would have been allowed to say that.' I appreciate this. People have done far better work than I have, know far more than I do, but they are not allowed to talk, and I happen to be."

But if the platform unquestionably helps, so does the effective talking of the man who mounts it. Burkitt is a nonstuffy talker—direct, simple, interesting, and amusing. And, despite their reputation otherwise, scientists like Burkitt's kind of talking and find it thought-provoking.

He uses slides, but hardly the usual dull kind. His are caricaturistic. He sketches them out and his daughter finishes them up for him. They illustrate his points and they are often very pointed points.

"I have been criticized," he says, "because I hold any brief for a hypothesis that would account for so many things detrimental to health even possibly resulting from the refining of foods. Much too simple, some say—too simple to have any chance of being right.

"But let's look at this slide, just a little diagram, showing a kettle standing on a table and a puddle of water standing beside the kettle. Now we can have different theories as to why there should be that puddle of water. One could be that steam from the kettle condenses on the handle, drips down the side of the kettle, and we have a little bit of a mess on the table. Quite popular.

"Another theory would have it that steam from the kettle goes up to the ceiling and condenses and the cold drops fall down on the kettle and drip down the side. And that is quite popular, too.

"And the last theory, which often may be overlooked, is that there simply may be a leak in the kettle.

"People," Burkitt goes on, "love to have complicated things. If somebody talks about something very complicated, they say, what a clever guy he is. You get somebody talking about psychology and he doesn't talk about 'instincts'; he talks about 'congenital hereditary predisposition,' and this sounds as if he knows all about it. A complicated name doesn't tell you anything more about a problem but it does hide our ignorance a bit."

Burkitt often uses a slide showing a dead elephant and a vulture. "This is a very important slide," he says. "In Africa, if you want to find a dead animal, you know that it will always be associated with vultures and scavengers. It is very hard to look for a dead animal by keeping your eyes on the ground and hunting in the grass. But if you look for vultures, they are easy to find. And when you find the vultures and then look down, there is the dead animal.

"Now you see," he says with a chuckle, "in medicine, we all tend to be either specialists in vultures or specialists in dead animals. So we don't look at the other thing. Yet, one disease may give you guidance about another, and relationships between diseases may suggest that they have a related cause or causes and may even give you a lead to which."

He has one slide he has used more than any other. "Here," he says, "you see water running out of a tap. The basin is full and the water is falling onto the floor. And there you see a couple of very hard-working, energetic, competent fellows whose aim in life is to try to keep the floor dry, mopping away constantly. But it has never occurred to them to turn off the tap.

"Now, the water running from the tap is like the cause of many diseases which may well be refined carbohydrates. The mess on the floor is like the diseases filling hospitals. And the men mopping away are like the doctors who take out gallbladders and appendixes and whatnot, but don't do anything about turning off the tap. There are two reasons for this. One is that the salary for the medical equivalent of floor mopping is about four times the salary for tap-turning-off. And the other thing is that industry is spending so much time making mops and brushes in the way of drugs and appliances and catgut and operating tables, and if we turned off the tap, you see, they would all be out of business."

Burkitt is not immune from being heckled. "Sometimes when I lecture," he says, "some bright guy will get up and say, I don't believe any of that stuff you are saying, Mr. Burkitt. And I say, fine—what is *your* hypothesis? Commonly, he will say, oh, I haven't done any thinking at all. And I will say, it is better to have a bad hypothesis than no hypothesis: you may be wrong but if you knock it down, you have gotten somewhere. When you are doing a jigsaw puzzle, you put together as many pieces of the puzzle as you can and then you set up a hypothesis as to what the pieces you have put together could possibly be part of. Because if you can imagine what the whole picture may be, it will be easier to put the remaining bits together.

"Now in this slide, the pieces that have been put together so far look like they might be part of the door, two windows, and back wheel of a carriage. So we hypothesize that the whole picture will be a carriage. But then we find a piece of the puzzle which doesn't fit in with the hypothesis. Now some researchers, when they find a fact that doesn't fit in with a hypothesis, throw the fact away. But you are not allowed to do that. It's dishonest. You have to say, sorry, I had the wrong hypothesis and have to begin again. So you need a new hypothesis. And you say, perhaps the completed jigsaw puzzle will show not a carriage but a little house, with a bicycle leaning against a wall. And now a piece that didn't fit into the picture of a carriage makes part of the roof of the house. And then you get all the other bits to fit in, and now your hypothesis has become a fact."

Always, Burkitt emphasized that the idea of refined carbohydrates as the cause of many diseases was hypothesis, not yet fact. But it was a useful hypothesis—something very worthwhile going on. It might have to be modified—conceivably it might even have to be abandoned—if, as more facts were accumulated, they did not fit in. But it was an extremely valuable incentive for getting more facts and even a guide as to what facts were needed.

And as he went around visiting mission and other hospitals, talking with individual physicians, addressing medical meetings, Burkitt built up his reporting network, and in Africa, India, England, the United States, and elsewhere sparked the creative interest of many investigators.*

* To arouse that interest fully, it was sometimes necessary for Burkitt to correct a mistaken notion, shared even by some otherwise knowledgeable medical scientists, that primitive peoples invariably die young—that there are "few white-haired Africans."

"It's rubbish," he pointed out. "Absolute baloney! The thing is, people often have misinterpreted the fact that there are higher death rates at young ages among

And as he went around, he also discovered that a number of people had actually been working on parts of the dietary fiber-disease relationship independently, without being very much or at all aware of one another's work, and some had made very valuable discoveries.

---

primitive peoples from infectious diseases—and, at times, from pure starvation—to mean that there are no elders among them. But there are, indeed, elders—plenty of them to be seen in African villages. Indeed, Dr. Walker has shown that if an African reaches the age of about forty-five or fifty, he has a better chance of reaching ninety than a white person."

6

The buried thesis, the prisoners in South Africa, the schoolboys in England

IN 1969 Burkitt was in East Africa, visiting hospitals, extending his network. He was also collecting stools, obtaining samples from people in different countries. He wanted to check on the influence of diet on bowel behavior. And in a hospital laboratory in Kampala where he went to weigh his collection, he met Dr. Ted Dimock who was there doing a blood count.

"Ah, Mr. Burkitt," said Dimock, introducing himself, "I was very interested in your talk yesterday about dietary fiber and intestinal disease. In the back ages, I did a thesis on this."

And, to Burkitt's astonishment, more than thirty years before, Ted Dimock had, in fact, weighed stools and made significant observations for his M.D. thesis at Cambridge, and the thesis and its findings had been buried on a shelf ever since and deserved resurrection.

Dimock was and is an unusual physician and man. All his medical life a country GP, he had, in 1966, once his family was raised, given up his practice to become a mission doctor in Uganda.

From the beginning of his medical career, he had been an iconoclast. Intestinal complaints were common, then as now. And it was common medical practice to prescribe special diets for such patients, diets that barred many foods, including fruits, which, it seemed to Dimock, were valuable. He intensely disliked—had a "horror" of—the purgation that was commonly employed by doctors and nurses for such patients, considering it medieval.

Cautiously at first, and then with increasing confidence, Dimock had begun to prescribe bran for his patients with constipation, those with vague abdominal complaints and what was often called "spastic colon," and patients with hemorrhoids. He wanted to use unprocessed bran, the untreated discard from milling, but it was not readily available then. He used a prepared bran cereal instead.

Bran then was called "roughage"—and even now is still called that by many. Dimock was irritated by the term; he did not regard it as roughage at all, and it struck him that a lot of medical nonsense was being taught.

Dimock was no academician. But a very good friend of his was. He had gone to Cambridge with Harry Himsworth and together they had trained at University College Hospital. At thirty Himsworth had become professor of medicine.

It was Himsworth who, upon hearing Dimock's views and learning that his friend was then successfully treating more than 300 patients with bran cereal, encouraged him to do a study on the effects on bowel behavior for an M.D. thesis at Cambridge.

For the study Dimock selected a group of patients with constipation, irritable colon, and other abdominal complaints. He obtained stool samples and he obtained further samples after putting the patients on bran.

He had no special facilities for his stool analyses. He had to carry them out at home and it was not a pleasant job. He carried them out at the bottom of his garden, well away from the house. Among other things, he weighed the stools, then used a little stove to heat and dehydrate them, and then weighed them again to see how much water they had contained. It took two to three hours on the stove and it was, he recalls, "a bit of a smelly job."

But Dimock found that with the use of bran, stool weights increased markedly and they were bulkier and softer, with more water in them. It was understandable that such stools could be passed more readily as compared to the small hard stools of the constipated and that their softness helped those with hemorrhoids. Somehow, too, with such stools, patients with spastic or irritable colon also benefited.

Hearing of the results, Harry Himsworth switched many of his patients onto bran and set about trying to eliminate purgation in wards. It was not easy. In 1936 Dimock wrote his thesis and also published a short paper in the British *Medical Journal* on his study. There was hardly an enthusiastic greeting for either.

"If you read the letters to the *Journal* after my paper," Dimock recalls, "they were very rude. And one of the doctors who examined me at Cambridge—I had to go through a cross-examination process by two physicians and defend my thesis—was astonished and miffed. 'You,' he exclaimed, 'would have me leave off my salts for my patients! Bosh!' But they granted my M.D. anyway."

But the thesis had remained in limbo for thirty-three years until Dimock got it off the shelf for Burkitt.

Far removed from Dimock and his thesis work in England, Burkitt was to discover that Dr. Alexander R. P. Walker in South Africa had done similar studies and had carried them further. Burkitt met him upon visiting the South African Institute of Medical Research in Johannesburg.

Alec Walker is a biochemist, a small, white-haired man, very quiet, very thoughtful—a Scotsman who was educated at the University of Bristol in England and emigrated to South Africa in 1938. He spent his whole working career in nutritional research and the conditions or diseases linked with nutritional insufficiency or excess.

Walker's studies of bowel behavior originated because of a wartime problem. During World War II South Africa was short of wheat. In wartime there is almost always a tendency to change from white bread to brown since for brown bread less bran is extracted and the wheat supply can go further.

In Britain, during the war, 85 percent extraction bread meal was used, with only 15 percent of the bran removed as against the usual 25 to 30 percent removal. In South Africa thought was given to going beyond what was considered to be Britain's halfway measure and using 95 to 100 percent extraction bread meal, discarding only 5 percent or less of the bran.

But there had been some concern in Britain that with higher extraction bread meal, less of the phytic acid in the meal would be removed, and phytic acid, with an affinity for calcium, might lessen the absorption of that important mineral. So in Britain calcium was added to the bread meal to counterbalance the greater ingestion of phytic acid. (And it is still being added even now to bread meal of lesser extraction as a kind of insurance policy.)

What then in South Africa? If 95 to 100 percent extraction meal was to be used, how much more calcium should be added?

It fell to Walker to carry out calcium balance studies in whites and Africans fed first on large amounts of white bread followed by large amounts of brown. In a balance study the intake of a material in food is compared with the output of it in urine and feces to determine how much if any is being retained.

Walker did the studies, many of them on African prisoners. He himself was one of the white subjects. He found that with a switch from white to brown bread, there were losses of calcium over the first month or so but then the losses became less and less. And not only was balance reached, but soon there were gains in calcium. Given time, the body adapted to the brown bread.

"Actually," Alec Walker says, "we felt that this must be the case. We couldn't think otherwise because unless the body has a mechanism of adaptation how could our forefathers have managed in regard to teeth and bones (for which calcium is essential) on their whole-grain cereals and brown bread diets?"

And it was in the course of carrying out these studies that Walker became intrigued by the evident difference in the bowel behavior between whites on the usual refined Western diet and the African prisoners who customarily received in prison their native high fiber diet.

One of the first things he noticed was the very large amount of feces passed per day by the Africans. Stool weights commonly were 150, 250, 350 grams for them, three times the weights for whites.

It was also striking that the Africans passed more than one stool a day; their average was more like two a day. In whites, the average is at best one a day.

There was another arresting difference. "We were intrigued," says Walker, "because we saw it before our eyes. In carrying out balance studies, we use a marker, a pill of carmine, a red dye. The dye is not absorbed but goes through the intestinal tract and comes out coloring the stool red. In balance studies we use the dye to relate a particular meal to a particular stool sample. We quickly became aware that the red pill was going through Bantu subjects much more rapidly than through white subjects. They were passing it in as little as nine hours and on average in one-third the time for white subjects. We thought surely all this taken together must have profound ramifications for the physiology of the African as compared with the physiology of the whites—and indeed in terms of pathology—of bowel conditions or diseases in Africans as compared with whites."

So Walker started to look into all of that. He began by querying prison doctors in many prisons in South Africa. They were consistent in indicating that, first of all, African prisoners had a very low prevalence of constipation; they seldom needed salts to help bowel motility. Secondly, the prison doctors reported, they found that appendicitis among these people was extremely rare. Walker himself, in taking a few samples of blood from Bantu prisoners, noticed that the cholesterol levels were low.

Walker began to check further. What about constipation and appendicitis in white prisoners? White prisoners do not consume the same type of diet inside prison as they do outside. They are not forced onto the native African diet served in prison but they do get a diet higher in brown bread, lower in fat, sugar, and meat than on the outside.

"The information we got from prison doctors and prison nurses," recalls Walker, "was that the necessity for purgatives among white prisoners was far less than outside. We learned that the incidence of appendicitis even in young prisoners—and the young are the most vulnerable to appendicitis—was much lower than in the general population outside prison. It also appeared that middle-aged prisoners who were diabetics required less insulin and many were able to do without, maintaining a low blood sugar merely on the prison diet."

Burkitt was impressed by Walker's work. He joined forces with him and with others now in determining daily stool weights and transit times (the times required for the remains of a meal to be excreted in the stool) in groups of various races in different countries. There were studies of children and adults in the United Kingdom, of Indian nurses in South India, of urban schoolchildren in South Africa, of rural South African schoolchildren, of rural villagers in Uganda, and of others.

Clearly, the more refined the diet, the smaller the stool and the slower the passage of food residues through the intestine. By contrast, diets containing ample fiber produce stools that are bulky, soft, and traverse the gut rapidly.

Then, with the guidance of Burkitt in organizing it, Dr. D. K. Payler of the Malvern Hospital in Worcestershire, England, undertook a simple study to determine what changes might be effected in bowel behavior by restoring fiber to a fiber-depleted diet.

Payler worked with nineteen boys, aged fifteen to nineteen years, in a boy's boarding school and two members of the school staff who agreed to serve as volunteer subjects. Average daily stool weights and intestinal transit times were measured while the subjects were on the normal school diet that included white bread. The transit times were found to vary between 22 and 157 hours with a mean of 64.5 hours or better than 2½ days. Daily stool weights were as low as 39 grams.

The volunteers were then given two heaping dessert spoonfuls of unprocessed miller's bran daily (about 14 grams) and were supplied with whole-meal bread instead of white (average two slices per day). After twenty-two days on the new diet, transit times and stool weights were again measured. The mean transit time dropped by 29 percent to 45.9 hours and the mean average of daily stool weight went up 21 percent to 163 grams.

Restoring fiber to the diet, Payler concluded, could do much to prevent constipation and might significantly alter bowel behavior toward that characteristic of people far less troubled or even free of bowel diseases common in civilized countries. "This simple expedient," he reported in the British medical journal *The Lancet,* "might well do more to 'keep the doctor away' than the proverbial apple."

Even as Payler was carrying out his study, a group of physicians at the Bristol Royal Infirmary were carrying out another and getting unexpected results.

Not at all to their surprise, the Bristol group found that adding fiber to the diet can help people with constipation—but they were surprised to find that the addition might well help people with nonspecific diarrhea (not associated with any specific infection or disease).

They worked with a group of twenty volunteers. They were all generally healthy. But twelve were bothered by either constipation or diarrhea. All were eating diets with a low content of fiber.

Transit times were measured and then the subjects ate either their normal diet supplemented with about 30 grams of unprocessed bran a day or a high fiber diet containing whole-meal bread. After at least four weeks, transit times were measured again.

Sure enough, the bran or a high fiber diet reduced transit times, which were initially three days or longer, benefiting the constipated. But, unexpectedly, the bran or the diet slowed the initially rapid one-day transit time in the patients with diarrhea.

What it came down to was this: with the dietary change, most subjects had a two-day transit whether their previous transit had been slow or fast. That suggested that in some way dietary fiber "normalizes" bowel behavior—and it supported the idea that foods from which fiber has been removed, such as white flour, induce abnormal bowel behavior.

7

The emerging gut picture

DR. WALKER had had his attention called to the phenomenon by the reports from prison doctors: appendicitis was rare among African prisoners and also among white prisoners. Yet, appendicitis is one of the commonest abdominal emergencies in Western countries, with better than 300,000 appendices removed annually in the United States alone.

Walker soon checked further. Gold-mining companies in South Africa are hardheaded. Native workers in the mines sign on for periods of up to eighteen months at a time. It is tough work. The companies see that they get all they want of their native diets and provide excellent hospital facilities—often better, Walker remarks, than what the white population outside of the mines has. The hospitals keep excellent records. And the information from the mine hospitals was that appendicitis is extremely rare.

The phenomenon was not confined to South African natives. Denis Burkitt could recall that in 1961, in connection with the work on Burkitt's lymphoma, he had visited more than fifty hospitals in East and Central Africa and had reviewed their operation registers. Operations for acute appendicitis were distinctly uncommon.

And now his reporting network of mission hospitals was confirming the rarity of appendicitis throughout rural Africa. Of the first twenty-five hospitals in East Africa reporting in, none saw more than three cases a year. Ten did not admit more than one.

Four senior doctors responsible for all the surgery in their hospitals had not seen a single case of appendicitis in thirty, twenty-eight, eighteen, and seventeen years respectively.

When Burkitt went back into the medical literature, he found a striking document. Half a century before, Dr. Arthur Rendle Short, who was a lecturer in physiology before holding the Chair of Surgery at Bristol University in England, had advanced a thoughtful argument in the British *Journal of Surgery,* suggesting that the main cause of appendicitis was the removal of much of the cellulose content (the term "dietary fiber" was unknown at that time) of food. He blamed in particular the growing popularity of white flour and demonstrated a relationship between the rapid increase in its consumption with the consequent decrease in the consumption of coarser flour, and the incidence of acute appendicitis in Britain and North America. Short had concluded that the steep rise in the incidence of appendicitis was more closely linked to the refining of grain than to any other known factor. His surgical charge of Clifton College and his close association with Muller's Orphanage, which cared for more than 1,000 children, enabled him to recognize the striking contrast between the prevalence of appendicitis in cake- and pastry-eating public schoolboys and its rarity among orphans fed on much coarser fare.

Studying scores of reports on appendicitis appearing over many decades in the medical literature, Burkitt could trace a pattern. In less developed communities virtually everywhere, appendicitis was a rarity; more and more, as those communities developed and shifted to Western refined diets, or as natives moved from the less developed to the more developed, appendicitis increased and became common.

In Khartoum the incidence increased twentyfold in thirty years. At the Mulago Hospital in Kampala, Uganda, the operative rate for appendicitis went up by more than twenty times between 1952 and 1969. At the Korle Bu Hospital in Accra, Ghana, there were less than 10 operations a year for appendicitis in the 1940s; by 1960 there were 70; by 1965, 145 and another 64 were treated conservatively. In Nairobi, Kenya, in 1937, in a series of 1,000 autopsies on Africans, only a single case of appendicitis was found; by the late 1960s more than 150 cases a year were being admitted for surgery. When Sudanese soldiers were attached to British battalions in North Africa during World War II, they shared British rations and promptly became much more liable to appendicitis than their compatriots on traditional Sudanese food.

And there was the striking change, too, in the appendicitis incidence among American blacks. In the early years of this century acute appendicitis was far less common among blacks than among whites. In New Orleans in the early 1930s blacks still had only one-fourth as much appendicitis as whites. By 1950, as their economic circumstances began to improve somewhat, appendicitis had become half as common among them as among whites. And the disparity has now almost disappeared and, in clearly similar economic circumstances as, for example, in the army, the incidence is comparable in both races.

But appendicitis hardly stood alone as a bowel disease common in advanced countries with refined diets and notably uncommon among peoples on unrefined diets.

In Britain and the United States diverticular disease has become the commonest disease of the large bowel, present in more than one-fifth of all over the age of forty, with the incidence rising far higher in the fifties, sixties, and later. Polyps of the colon have been reported present in one-third of all autopsies on patients over the age of twenty years. Cancer of the colon is, after lung cancer, the most common cause of death from cancer. In the United States alone, it affects 76,000 new patients each year and causes 46,000 deaths annually. Ulcerative colitis is also uncomfortably much too common, with a known prevalence of 80 per 100,000 population in Britain.

In sharp contrast, in all the communities where appendicitis is indigenously rare or absent, all of these other diseases of the bowel are even less common.

In twenty years of surgical practice in Uganda, Burkitt had never once seen a case of diverticular disease in an African. Even now, his network reports indicated that it was a rare disease in rural Africans. Of the first fifty-two mission hospitals reporting, forty-four had not recorded a single case of diverticular disease. Six others had recorded one case only. The remaining two had more cases but not many more. And a South African study of 2,367 autopsies on Bantu patients found only one case of diverticular disease.

Polyps of the colon and cancer of the colon and rectum are also rare in rural Africa. In a thirteen-year study of all autopsies and biopsies in a 2,500-bed South African hospital, only six polyps were found. Records for four separate rural areas in East Africa indicate that cancer of the colon and rectum accounts for as little as 1.1 percent of all cancers as against 12 percent in England.

The first case of ulcerative colitis ever reported in East or Central Africa, Burkitt found, was seen only in 1966.

Burkitt also determined that in Japan all these conditions had been rare until the last war, but with increasing use of Western diets were becoming more common. It had become apparent, too, that among Japanese migrating to Hawaii or California, the appendicitis rate soon became the same as that of the white population—and among these immigrants, diverticular disease became 3½ times as common as in Japan and colon cancer seven times as common. In a single generation, figures showed, the Japanese caught up 75 percent of the way to the white population's rate of colorectal cancer.

It was notable, too, that in Puerto Rico, as the Western type of diet became increasingly popular, the incidence of bowel cancer rose steadily.

And again, as with appendicitis, there was the experience of American blacks with bowel cancer. In the African villages from which their ancestors came, the malignancy remained almost unknown. Even fifty years ago, when the menus of black and white America differed markedly, bowel cancer affected two American whites for every black. Now, with little if any difference in diets, bowel cancer rates have equalized.

By 1972 Burkitt had obtained information from more than two hundred hospitals in over twenty countries. The information confirmed that appendicitis, diverticular disease of the colon, and both polyps and tumors of the colon are rare in the developing countries.

From these sources and others as well, he found that in no country or region is one of these diseases common and the others rare save that appendicitis, which afflicts the young, appears about a generation before the other conditions.

Consistently, too, he and Dr. Walker and other co-workers had found that in no community consuming a high fiber diet was any of these bowel diseases common, nor was there any community that had changed from a high to low fiber diet that had not become increasingly subject to most if not all of the conditions within a generation, with appendicitis heralding the advent of its companion diseases.

But how could the change in diet account for three such diverse conditions as appendicitis, diverticular disease, and cancer of the colon?

As Cleave saw it, diverticular disease arose because of excessive contractions of the colon. The contractions raised pressure within the colon, and eventually the pressure forced the inner mucous membrane lining of the colon through the muscular wall of the colon, producing little outpouchings.

He envisioned a simple sequence of events. On a refined diet the passage of feces through the large intestine slowed. Trying to move the material along, the colon contracted excessively. And there followed the elevated pressure and the diverticula formation. And in the United States in 1949, at the University of Chicago, Dr. Anton J. Carlson, often called the "grand old man" of physiology, found that while a low residue diet encouraged the formation of diverticula in rats, the addition of roughage prevented their development.

But what of appendicitis?

Man carries vestiges of his prehuman past—among them, body hair, wisdom teeth, fused tail vertebrae, muscles that move his ears, and the vermiform appendix. Whatever function the vermiform appendix (vermiform meaning wormlike) served in the past, it has no known use now.

The vestigial organ is a blind alley appended to the large intestine. Its length may be anywhere from less than an inch to nine inches, but generally it is just a bit over three inches. The appendix shares the fecal contents of a cul-de-sac pouch, which forms the first part of the colon or large intestine. Any fecal material that flows into the appendix normally is dumped right back into the pouch, which is known as the cecum.

But if the opening to the appendix should become blocked by a fecalith, a stony concretion that may form around a piece of fecal matter, appendicitis—inflammation—may follow, and if the appendix is not removed it may perforate and produce peritonitis, infection in the abdominal cavity.

That has been the general picture. But many investigators have long considered that raised pressures are important in producing appendicitis. Almost at the turn of the century one researcher had shown that increased pressures interfered with blood circulation in the mucous lining of the bowel. In the 1930s the famed American surgeon Dr. O. H. Wangensteen had shown experimentally that sustained pressures even for as little as six hours were followed by changes in the wall of the appendix.

Cleave had suggested that when fiber in the diet is reduced, sugar intake is increased and so, along with raised pressures in the colon and the slowing of feces passage as the result of the reduced fiber, the increased sugar led to a change in the bacterial colonies in the gut, encouraging the multiplication of highly infective organisms. Thus, the mucous lining, its circulation impaired by pressures, was more vulnerable to infection, and there were the highly infective organisms ready to pounce.

Burkitt did not believe that any change in the bacterial colonies in the colon had to be involved. If such a change did occur, it might be a contributory factor. He considered pressure to be the fundamental cause. By leading to devitalizing changes in the mucous membrane lining, it rendered the lining susceptible to invasion, and many of the naturally present bacteria could do the invading.

But how could refined diet account for cancer of the colon?

There could be many other possible reasons and, indeed, many had been considered by investigators. In his quiet, thorough way, Alec Walker had looked into them, studying very carefully the work that had been done to try to find a tenable explanation.

A first possibility, of course, is that the diet of people more prone to colon cancer might contain higher concentrations of carcinogens, or cancer-producing agents. They might operate in conjunction with—or even independently of—any intestinal problems.

Food additives might conceivably be the culprits. In most Western countries for many years food additives have been subjected to intensive tests. Yet, in practice, dietary carcinogens are difficult to detect in everyday diets.

Still, it was noteworthy that Denmark has one of the highest death rates in the world from colonic cancer despite extremely stringent regulations on food additives. Moreover, in India, a study in 1967 had shown that colonic cancer incidence varied greatly in various regions even though the populations in these regions had relatively little exposure to sophisticated modern food additives. Since there was no positive proof of a significant role for additives, other possibilities obviously deserved examination.

It might be that some particular food component was involved. High fat intake had come under suspicion. Some American investigators thought it might well be involved. So did some workers elsewhere. In 1969 in Czechoslovakia researchers had reported finding what seemed to be a high correlation between deaths from colonic cancer and the amount of animal protein consumed—and, of course, animal meats often contained sizable quantities of fat.

Yet, account had to be taken of the fact that American Indians in the Southwest consumed large amounts of fat, and they were not characterized by a high prevalence of colonic cancer. And the same was true of the Masai tribe in Africa, despite a strange diet composed almost entirely of huge quantities of meat, milk, and animal blood. It seemed unlikely to Walker that a single staple foodstuff or nutrient consumed in excess could be specifically noxious.

He could see a third and overlapping possibility: that the diets of people prone to colonic cancer might be associated with higher concentrations of carcinogenic metabolites or breakdown products with cancer-activating potential that were produced during their passage through the intestinal tract. And their noxiousness could depend largely, if not wholly, on intestinal conditions.

Burkitt could, did, and continues to build up a case for the striking influence of the intestinal conditions brought about by dietary fiber lack.

He took into account a whole series of studies, including some in 1969 and 1971, by many researchers. They had produced many facts that constituted pieces of evidence. These had to be accommodated and he could accommodate them.

The studies had shown that stools from areas with a high incidence of bowel cancer, such as England and North America, have a different bacterial content than those from low incidence areas such as Africa and Japan.

They had shown too that some of the strains of bacteria present in greater numbers in Western stools can act on bile salts that come into the gut from the liver and gallbladder to aid in the digestion of fats—and their activity on the bile salts could lead to the formation of products, chemical substances, known to be potentially carcinogenic.

Some of the researchers who had carried out these studies believed that it was the increased fat in Western diets that altered the bacterial composition, making for greater numbers of organisms capable of degrading bile salts. They argued, too, that a high intake of fat also meant that more bile salts poured into the bowel because they were needed for fat digestion, thus increasing the concentration of the salts in the feces. Thus, fats could, in effect, be double culprits.

Possibly so, Burkitt would grant.

But, *whether or not fat is a responsible dietary constituent,* the slowdown of fecal passage, the markedly increased transit time, that resulted from a low fiber diet was very much involved. With the slow movement of the feces, there was more time for the bacteria to proliferate in the stool and degrade the bile salts. Moreover, since the fecal mass with a low fiber diet was small, that meant a higher concentration of the carcinogens formed. And, on top of this, since the stool moved slowly, the carcinogens were retained for long periods against the intestinal lining, giving them prolonged time in which to stir up a malignant reaction.

Contact between feces and bowel lining seems to be essential for the production of colonic cancer, Burkitt could argue. For in animal studies, when the fecal stream was bypassed through an artificial detour around a section of bowel, cancer could develop elsewhere in the bowel but did not develop around the isolated segment.

Burkitt could also point to the fact that in areas where colonic cancer is common, it occurs mainly in the far or lower end of the colon. That would certainly be expected if some cancer-causing agent were produced during passage of the feces through the large bowel and would act most powerfully where stool slowdown and even arrest is greatest, as it is at the lower end of the colon.

An influence of lack of dietary fiber on the development of colonic cancer was consistent with the fact that where the malignancy had high prevalence so did appendicitis and diverticular disease, with all three uncommon in communities where dietry fiber intake was high but common where the intake was low. And it was also, importantly, consistent with the facts about two other worrisome diseases of the colon: polyps and ulcerative colitis.

The relationship between colonic cancer and adenomatous polyps (adenomatous meaning a tumor of the epithelium, the covering of internal and external surfaces of the body) is so close that many authorities consider them to be merely different manifestations of the same disease. Not only is their geographical distribution almost identical, but they have a similar anatomical distribution in the colon and rectum, a similar age distribution, and they tend to be associated in the same individuals. The relationships are so close that some common causative factor or factors must be operating. It seems likely to Burkitt—and now to many other investigators—that if degraded products of bile salts are in part responsible for malignant tumors, they may also cause benign adenomatous polyp growths. And the concentration of these products and the prolonged exposure of them to the intestinal wall by small slow-moving stools characteristic of low fiber intake may be very much involved.

Ulcerative colitis is one of man's nastiest afflictions. A disease of young adulthood and the middle years, it can produce bloody, uncontrolled diarrhea with as many as fifteen to thirty bowel movements a day, with anemia, fever, emaciation, and prostration. It can be a life-threatening disorder. Involved in it are inflammatory changes that make the intestine appear red, swollen, and in some areas ulcerated.

In victims of ulcerative colitis, cancer of the colon occurs more frequently and at younger ages. And the frequent association between ulcerative colitis and cancer has usually been explained on the basis that somehow the inflammatory, ulcerative process is transformed into a malignant process.

Yet, the explanation fails to account for the fact that other chronic ulcerative conditions in the bowel—those, for example, produced by infection with amoeba (amebiasis) or by infection with flat, wormlike organisms known as Schistosoma flukes (schistosomiasis)—show no tendency to malignant change. Nor is there any other known human inflammatory lesion that frequently is transformed into a malignancy. Everything considered, it appears to Burkitt and other researchers now that cancer of the colon and ulcerative colitis may well have a common cause and that lack of dietary fiber logically could be it.

When, not long ago, Burkitt—because of his studies on colonic cancer and its association with other diseases of the colon—was asked to write an editorial for the *Journal* of the U.S. National Cancer Institute, he chose to do so on the subject of "Some Neglected Leads to Cancer Causation."

In it he noted how the association of colonic cancer with other colon diseases and of the latter with dietary fiber intake had suggested what seemed to him to be a very likely factor, a major one, in the bowel malignancy.

And he went on then to wonder whether cancer research might sometimes be too "blinkered" because of a tendency to focus only on malignant lesions to the exclusion of other conditions, "the investigation of which might point the way to a better understanding of certain forms of cancer."

True, he remarked, there had been enormous and expensive development of tools and techniques to explore constructions and mechanisms deep within tiny single cells, but "there has been perhaps neglect of the wider view that sees cancer within the context of other associated diseases."

8

Mr. Painter and the complete reversal

SO far so good. A hypothesis is a useful device. It is not itself a truth or a fact. Rather, it is a tentative theory or supposition adopted because it seems to explain certain facts and because it may serve as a guide in the investigation of others.

Denis Burkitt has always emphasized this about the hypothesis that dietary change—the shift to refined foods and the resulting loss of dietary fiber—may be responsible, in whole or in part, for many diseases and disturbances.

A hypothesis is not even the equivalent of a theory, let alone a law. Hypothesis implies that there is evidence that a principle is operating but more evidence is desirable, and so what the hypothesis offers is a tentative explanation. A theory implies a much greater range of evidence and greater likelihood of truth. A law implies a statement of order and relation that has been found to be invariable under the same conditions.

A hypothesis needs to be subjected to practical testing. And it was a surgeon in a London hospital who subjected it to some particularly vigorous testing.

Neil Painter took a hard—and internal—look at diverticular disease. He actually measured and took pictures of what happens in the colon. He went on then to treatment of the disease, treatment diametrically opposed to the conventional treatment, and, because of his successes, within the last three or four years treatment on a worldwide basis has swung around 180 degrees. And, beyond that, his work was to throw light on the origin of many very common but ill-defined and unexplained "bellyaches" lumped under such labels as "spastic colon," "irritable colon," and "irritable bowel syndrome."

Neil Painter, now senior surgeon at Manor House Hospital in Golders Green, London, came to medicine late. A navy pilot in World War II, he entered medical school at the age of twenty-three and qualified at twenty-nine. He went on then to further training. He wanted to work for an M.S. degree; it would be helpful, he considered, in furthering his career, aiding in the competition to obtain a surgical consultancy. At Oxford in 1960 he looked around for some research to do that could be applied to obtaining the M.S.

Just at that time Oxford had acquired a machine for measuring pressures in the colon. It was being used as an aid in studying the normal physiology of the colon.

No one, Painter soon found, had ever measured colonic pressures in diverticular disease. He was fascinated by the disease because of its curious history.

Colonic diverticula, or outpouchings, had been described a century before when it was far from common. There had even been some belief among a few scientists that the condition might result from constipation, which caused some form of obstruction. But diverticula were regarded as harmless curiosities until the turn of the century when one physician suggested that they might lead to peritonitis and other lethal complications.

The disease was so new that even by 1920 it had not yet found its way into medical textbooks. But by 1930 diverticula were being found in about 5 percent of colons of people over forty. And thirty years later, the disease, almost unknown in 1900, had become the commonest abnormality of the colon in the Western world, with studies in the United States, the United Kingdom, Australia, and France showing that between one-third and one-half of those over forty have diverticula, and the incidence rises to two-thirds at later ages.

To do his measuring, Painter used three open-ended, fine, water-filled tubes, each only 2 millimeters in diameter. They could be introduced without great difficulty into the colon through the rectum and, with the ends of the tubes spaced 7.5 millimeters apart, Painter could pick up pressures at three levels in the colon. The pressures were transmitted through the water in the tubes to a transducer, which converted them so they could be read on a meter.

Painter coupled his pressure recordings with X-ray movies of the colon. And with the combination of the two, he found that the normal colon produces waves of pressure that are usually less than 10 millimeters of mercury in amplitude. The pressure changes are brought about by small movements of the walls of the colon, which act to propel the fecal stream along. And when there is no resistance to the movement of the walls other than that offered by the viscosity of the intestinal contents—which is not great resistance—the pressure changes are not great.

But it is another story, Painter found, in a patient who for many years has had small hard stools. Such stools call for an entirely different action by the colon. Where, with normal, soft, bulky stools—they can be likened somewhat, Painter says, to soft toothpaste—the colon walls need not contract much to assure passage and the pressures are small, when the stools are small and hard, the colon walls must contract harder, clamping down. There are contracting rings spaced along the walls and as these clamp down hard, they momentarily close down the colonic passageway, with chambers of high pressure formed between the contracting rings.

And it is the high pressures—Painter's measurements showed them reaching in excess of 90 millimeters of mercury—between the contracting rings that cause trouble. In effect, a chamber between two rings is obstructed momentarily at both ends and pressure builds up within it in much the same way as the urinary bladder can generate pressure and become painful when its outflow is obstructed.

The high pressure impinges on the mucous membrane lining of the colon wall. It pushes very hard on the lining and eventually it extrudes the lining, pushes it through the muscular segments of the colon wall, and herniates it.

In the course of his studies Painter experimented with many things. Drugs sometimes were used to try to relieve the pain of acute diverticular disease. Morphine was one of them. But Painter showed that, although in other situations morphine might be a potent analgesic, it was worse than useless in diverticular disease because it acted to increase the number and strength of pressure waves. On the other hand, he found that Demerol, a fairly potent analgesic, had the reverse effect on the pressures and might serve far better than morphine.

Painter also experimented with agents to soften up the feces and add bulk to it. Normacol was one such agent—a gum that absorbs water in the gut, swells up, and forms a bulky, watery stool.

He also considered diet. Checking into any research that might have been done previously, Painter found that in 1949 a radiological study carried out by an English doctor had indicated that the colons of Africans were wide bore, and had suggested that this might be due to the bulky diet they used.

Painter did some studies with rats. Those fed a diet lacking in fiber developed small, contracted colons with diverticular disease; those fed a high fiber diet did not.

From everything he had done, it seemed to Painter that there was a very good case for lack of dietary fiber being a prime factor in the development of diverticular disease.

Could the restoration of fiber help patients who already had the disease? He could not be certain. But the very idea went against all the standard, long-accepted medical teaching: do just the reverse for diverticular disease—avoid all "roughage" for that could only irritate and exacerbate the condition.

And yet Painter knew that by the early 1960s some physicians had gone off the no-roughage kick because it simply did not work and were telling patients to eat what they liked. They had not gone beyond that, had not given any thought to the possibility that a high residue diet might help. That would be an extreme 180-degree swing.

But the more Painter considered it, the more he thought it worth trying. He had become aware of Cleave's use of unprocessed bran for constipation, for Cleave, hearing of Painter's work, had been in touch with him about his own experience. Cleave had seen no complications from the use of bran in relieving constipation. In his checking Painter also learned about Dimock's work with prepared bran cereal for spastic colon as well as constipation, and Dimock had established its safety.

Painter decided to try a high fiber diet—beginning very cautiously with just a few patients. And when he began to see some evidence of value and none of harm, he undertook a full-scale study. He started it in December 1967, and carried on with it through 1971. Cleave encouraged him. In the course of the study, too, he met and became associated with Denis Burkitt whose detailed findings about the distribution of diverticular disease around the world and its rarity among peoples with high fiber diets further encouraged him.

By May 1971, Painter was reviewing, with Burkitt, the problem of diverticular disease as a deficiency disease of Western civilization in a major paper in the *British Medical Journal,* with some mention of the gratifying results he was getting in his treatment trial. A year later, in the same journal, with the treatment trial concluded, Painter wrote a full report of it, which was to have major beneficial repercussions around the world.

For the trial Painter and his associates at Manor House Hospital —Dr. Anthony Z. Almeida, also a surgeon, and Dr. Kenneth W. Colebourne, a physician—worked with seventy patients with diverticular disease. These were carefully checked to make as certain as possible that they had no cancer or disease other than diverticular.

The patients were put on what, for the sake of brevity, was called the "bran diet." There was much more to it than bran. It was a high dietary fiber diet. Patients were advised to eat bran cereal, porridge, whole-meal bread, fruits, and vegetables, and to reduce their intake of refined sugar. They were also told to take two teaspoons of unprocessed bran, which Painter got in large lots direct from a miller. They were to take that amount three times a day, and they were to increase the dose if necessary after two weeks until their bowels were open once or twice a day, without straining. They were warned that they might experience some flatulence, but that this would be temporary. The correct dosage of bran would be found by trial and error. Those who did not tolerate bran were advised to take a high residue diet supplemented by Normacol.

Of the 70 patients, 45 were men aged thirty-seven to eighty-two, and 25 were women aged thirty-six to seventy-eight.

The amount of bran needed to prevent straining at stool varied greatly, probably because the amount of fiber in the rest of each patient's diet, and hence its degree of fiber depletion, varied considerably. The bran requirement ranged from one dessert spoon daily (3 grams) to three tablespoons three times a day (45 grams). On average, two teaspoons three times a day—about 12 to 14 grams —made stools soft and easy to pass.

Unprocessed bran is difficult to eat dry and no patient tried to eat it that way. Most sprinkled it on cereal, some took it with milk or water, a few added it to soup. No fewer than thirty-nine patients felt distended and suffered from flatulence when they first took the bran. Usually, flatulence disappeared within three weeks but in some cases lasted for eight weeks. In three patients a sensation of slight distention persisted but they preferred it to their previous symptoms.

Eight patients did not take bran. Several felt nauseated or too distended by it to continue. A few preferred Normacol instead. Three were so improved by eating whole-meal bread, a prepared bran cereal, and other fiber in the diet that they stopped taking the unprocessed bran and remained comfortable.

Bowel habits changed dramatically. Not only did constipated patients pass soft motions regularly but those who formerly passed frequent small stools or had attacks of diarrhea had fewer but soft-formed motions. Before the diet the majority of patients had strained at stool virtually all the time and a number of others did so frequently. With the diet fifty-one said straining at stool was a thing of the past. Most of the patients reported that they now emptied their bowels completely whereas before this was not the case.

Patients with diverticular disease may complain of several symptoms. Altogether, the total of symptoms for the 70 patients was 171, an average of about 2½ per patient.

One or more dyspeptic symptoms—nausea, heartburn, flatulence, distension, wind—were common. Lower or general abdominal pain occurred in 28 patients, 29 had localized pain or ache elsewhere, and 12 had severe colic. Tender rectum, incomplete emptying of rectum, and constipation afflicted many.

With the change in diet symptoms were relieved in 88.6 percent of the patients. Nausea, heartburn, flatulence, distension, and wind; pain, ache, and severe colic; constipation and the rest—all responded, either being relieved or often abolished. One patient who had defecated twelve times a day and another who had done so six times a day passed motions only twice a day on the diet.

The majority of the patients had taken laxatives. Only seven felt they needed laxatives once on the diet. The diet did not change the appetite of patients whose appetite was good but improved it in twenty-six whose appetite had been poor.

In not one case was the appetite made worse by the diet. "This," says Painter, "suggests that the widely held view that so-called 'roughage' irritates the gut is not founded on fact; bran when moist becomes 'softage.' "

Painter likes to note particularly the twelve cases of severe colic because when diverticular disease becomes that painful patients often have come to surgery. None has had to go to surgery.

When he learned of Painter's work, Adam Smith, a distinguished Scottish surgeon, became interested in what possibilities a high fiber diet might have from another standpoint. Smith is a reader in surgery—the equivalent in the United States of professor and head of the department—at the University of Edinburgh. His department is a special one, a gastrointestinal unit devised to enable patients with bowel diseases of all sorts to be treated in an area staffed by doctors representing many medical and surgical specialties, who could work jointly when that was necessary to help an individual patient.

A major concern of Smith, as a surgeon, and of the whole department, was to try to learn more about gastrointestinal physiology, including more that could be helpful when surgery became necessary. It was a fact of life in surgery that an operation might produce benefits in some conditions but the benefits did not last long. Patients soon had recurrences of their old problems.

Diverticular disease was one of these. Two types of operation for the disease could be used. In one, resection, a length of large bowel affected by the disease was removed and the remaining portions of the bowel were drawn together and sutured. In the other, a more recent development known as myotomy, the surgeon does not remove any of the colon but instead makes an incision along the length of an affected section, splitting the outer coats of muscle in the colon wall, to allow the wall to relax.

With either operation for a time there might be significant benefits but they were not permanent. Smith and his associates set out to determine why.

It now appeared that high pressures within the colon are involved in producing diverticular disease. They also knew that the pressures were brought about by colonic motility, the vigorousness with which the walls of the colon contracted.

If they measured the motility, that could also give them indications of the pressure. And they could measure the motility by introducing multiple balloons into the lower colon and, with the balloons connected to recording equipment, they could record the motility both before and after it was stimulated by food or by a drug such as neostigmine.

They made such measurements in patients before and after surgery. They found that in patients after the myotomy operation there was a considerable reduction in intestinal motor activity in response to both food and neostigmine compared to what had prevailed before surgery. But the resection patients demonstrated no such reduction, indicating that the abnormality in diverticular disease is generalized and not affected by removing a length of colon, although there might be some immediate relief of symptoms.

But the encouraging fall in motility after myotomy, it soon became evident, only lasted for about a year, after which it started to climb again and within two to three years was back to what it had been before surgery. Thus, neither surgical procedure provided definitive treatment.

It was about this time that Smith met Neil Painter at a medical meeting. It was well before Painter's study using a high fiber diet was completed, but Painter could give him early highly encouraging information about the value of the diet in nonsurgical treatment of diverticular disease.

Smith and his associates promptly decided to study the effect on patients after surgery. They put patients, soon after operation, on a daily dose of 20 grams of unprocessed bran in addition to their regular diet.

The results were startling. Among patients who had undergone resection of the colon and therefore would be expected to show little if any reduction at all in colon motility, there was and has continued to be, during the five years the study in Edinburgh has been in progress, a considerable and well-maintained reduction. And among patients who had undergone myotomy and showed as usual an initial reduction in motor activity, the motility has not shot back up again during the five years.

"Indeed," says Adam Smith, "the colonic activity fell even lower than it did with myotomy alone and has been well maintained. In view of our findings, we advise giving patients bran after either a resection or myotomy."

And Painter agrees. To him, if surgery has to be used, it is only an "incident" in treatment. "If the cause of diverticular disease is to be removed, the patient must not return to his former fiber-deficient diet."

Painter's observations in connection with his studies of the use of a high fiber diet in diverticular disease are having repercussions and promise to have even more that go beyond that disease alone.

There is, he points out, double significance in the fact that such a diet relieves the symptoms of diverticular disease. For the relief is achieved even though the diverticula, the outpouchings, remain.

So the symptoms cannot be due to the diverticula. Where, then, can they stem from?

Well, consider, suggests Painter: If a fiber-deficient diet can damage the colon enough to produce diverticula, it has to be extremely unlikely that the colon, and often only one region of it (the sigmoid), is the only part of the gut adversely affected by a fiber-deficient diet. The symptoms could well originate in other parts of the gut that also have not adapted to a low residue diet and whose motility is altered by this diet.

And the concept that the whole of the gastrointestinal tract has to struggle with a low residue diet, Painter points out, explains not only why such "upper intestinal" symptoms as nausea and heartburn accompany diverticulosis but also how a high fiber diet relieves them.

Even more than that, Painter is convinced that this concept may also throw some light on the origin of the symptoms of "spastic colon," "irritable colon," and "irritable bowel syndrome."

"These are ill-defined conditions and are used as convenient terms to account for the presence of any unexplained 'bellyache,'" says Painter, a husky but gentle gray-haired man given to speaking softly but trenchantly.

"The 'irritable bowel syndrome' is said to be responsible for the symptoms of up to 60 percent of patients attending gastrointestinal clinics in whom no abnormality of the alimentary tract can be demonstrated."

(The symptoms are extremely variable: abdominal distress is common and may take the form of generalized abdominal distention, cramps, sharp knifelike pains, or deep dull pain. Other common complaints include nausea, heartburn, excessive belching, constipation or diarrhea or one alternating with the other. And some patients complain as well of weakness, headaches, faintness, and excessive perspiration.)

"Now the term 'irritable bowel syndrome'—and the other terms of 'spastic colon' and 'irritable colon' often used interchangeably with it—implies that these 60 percent of patients have abnormal alimentary tracts. But," says Painter, "on evolutionary grounds, it is extremely unlikely that such a high proportion of the population is born with a congenitally abnormal intestine."

A better term, Painter suggests, would be "irritated (rather than irritable) bowel syndrome." That would connote what would be nearer to the truth: that the bowel is not abnormally irritable but rather is being abnormally irritated.

"Such a change of emphasis in our thinking," he tells the medical profession, "would be of the greatest importance. Normal intestinal tracts would no longer be blamed for symptoms that are almost certainly caused by our overrefined modern diet. We might then retrace our dietary footsteps with the result that future generations would not develop diverticulosis or suffer from those other diseases of the colon that presently afflict our citizens."

When I saw Neil Painter at Manor House Hospital not long ago, he told me with a chuckle: "It may well be that a lot of the symptoms listed in the medical textbooks under various abdominal diseases are really general gut symptoms due to Western diet. Remember the textbooks were written after technology refined our food. It could, indeed, well be that a lot of the textbook symptoms are nonspecific and really have nothing to do with the diseases to which they are attributed. This is something I'm trying to find time to work on and I think it will upset quite a few people."

Already, of course, Painter has upset the old dictum about treating diverticular disease, with many physicians in England, the United States, and elsewhere now switched from having their patients avoid "roughage" as an "irritant" and instead consuming a high fiber diet as a means of removing the irritant effects of a refined low fiber diet.

And his recent report that symptoms of so-called "irritable bowel syndromes" also often respond to a high fiber diet may also be beginning to stir up a useful upset.

Already, Painter's results in treating that syndrome have very recently been confirmed in the United States by Dr. Joseph L. Piepmeyer, a medical officer in the U.S. Naval Reserve stationed at Beaufort, North Carolina, Naval Hospital. In a study he did with thirty patients with irritable bowel symptoms, Piepmeyer prescribed eight to ten teaspoons of bran a day for three weeks. Four patients dropped out because they found the bran unpalatable. But twenty-three of the twenty-six who used the bran, 88 percent, reported improvement in their symptoms.

9

. . . and some matters of great strain

NEIL PAINTER had noticed it. Among his patients with diverticular disease, some had suffered with hemorrhoids. Several had first-degree hemorrhoids or piles, symptomatic, bleeding a bit, painful. Others had second-degree piles, with prolapse and very big dilated veins.

Often, after they were placed on a high fiber diet and once their motions became soft as a result of the diet, not only their diverticular disease symptoms improved. They did well with their hemorrhoids, which stopped bleeding and no longer were painful.

"The veins were still dilated," Painter says. "Whether, over a period of time without constipation and straining at stool, they will settle down, I don't know. But the patients are comfortable."

He recalls one patient—"an old dear who, along with diverticular disease, had piles and a hiatus hernia, too. She had been damned uncomfortable. But on the diet for more than three years—she was one of those in the trial and we followed them all closely—she was fine in every department.

"Does it seem that everything responds to high fiber?" Painter remarks with a chuckle. "We mustn't oversell. That 'old dear' with all those things . . . give her bran and she is better. Fine. To say that lack of fiber might be the cause of all her problems could be too much. But fiber helps. And it is a fact that many problems go together in the civilized world and perhaps many of them have something in common in the way of a cause."

Hemorrhoids, varicose veins, and deep vein thrombosis—three

blood vessel diseases that seem in no way connected with the gastrointestinal tract—are all significant problems in Western countries, and the last is often a deadly one. Denis Burkitt was to spend a good deal of study establishing that they could, in fact, share a common causative factor, alterations in intestinal behavior.

Varicose veins and hemorrhoids—both of them conditions in which veins become dilated and engorged, in the one case in the legs and in the other inside or just outside the rectum—are among the most common ailments of economically developed countries. Recent studies suggest that in many Western countries the frequency of varicose veins in adults approximates 50 percent. Hemorrhoids are even more common.

Deep vein thrombosis is the grave problem. A thrombus, or blood clot, forms in a deep vein in the leg. The clot lengthens out to produce a kind of freely waving tail. As the clot also increases in diameter, it obstructs the vein. A deep vein thrombosis can lead to swelling, pain, or tenderness of the leg. Eventually, the clot may stop growing and become firmly attached to the vein wall and, over a period of months, the body, responding to the blockage of the vein, may form new vessel pathways to bypass the blocked area.

But a major danger is that at some point during the time when the clot is not firmly attached to the vein wall, part or all of it may break loose, travel rapidly in the bloodstream, and end up lodged in and blocking a major lung vessel. Then, it is a pulmonary embolism, a dreaded disaster, which may take life and does in fact kill about 2,500 people in Britain annually and many thousands more in the United States.

Deep vein thrombosis is common in surgical patients. An American study in 1970 found it occurring in from 20 to 30 percent of all patients undergoing surgery and in 40 to 45 percent of all older patients undergoing major operations. It is no less common in severe medical illness. Two British studies established that it occurs in about 35 percent of hospitalized medical patients over the age of forty.

And pulmonary embolism resulting from deep vein thrombosis is now responsible for as many as 9 percent of all deaths occurring in hospitals.

From his own experience, from information supplied by his network of reporting mission hospitals, and from other data, Burkitt soon was establishing that the geographical distribution of varicose veins and deep vein thrombosis is almost identical—and that the distribution of hemorrhoids is similar, with the hemorrhoid incidence rising in any community before that of varicose veins.

All three conditions proved to be common in economically developed communities but rare in all developing countries and almost unknown in tribal communities where the influence of Western countries is slight. Where Western dietary customs have been adopted over recent years—as in urban Africa, for example—the diseases were increasing in incidence.*

---

* Burkitt himself could recall that in 1962 he had examined more than 4,000 adults during a sleeping sickness inspection in one of the less developed areas of Central Africa and had found only five cases of varicose veins, an incidence of 0.12 percent—about 1/1,000th of the incidence in Great Britain.

In 1971 one of his corresponding physicians set out to look specifically for varicose veins for more than a year in a hospital dealing annually with some 30,000 outpatients, members of a tribe in Africa still almost unaffected by Western civilization. He found only one case.

That same year another corresponding physician, in an area somewhat more developed in Malawi, found an incidence of about 0.2 percent in recruits for work in the South African mines. When Burkitt sent out questionnaires to mission hospitals in 20 countries in sub-Saharal Africa, 89 estimated that they saw fewer than five patients with varicose veins annually. And inquiries at 33 mission hospitals in India and Pakistan showed that 16 had seen fewer than five patients annually and only five had seen more than 20 cases.

Not only varicose veins but hemorrhoids as well proved to be rare throughout rural Africa and almost unknown in the more primitive communities. At the Charles Johnson Memorial Hospital in Zululand, during a three-year period in which over 11,000 patients were admitted and more than 100,000 outpatients seen, only a single case of hemorrhoids was noted.

It also turned out—for both varicose veins and hemorrhoids—that where the incidence is now rising, it is in the urban population, adopting Western ways. Among the reports Burkitt received from corresponding physicians was one from Dr. C. G. Bremner at the Baragwanath Hospital in Johannesburg. There, between 1960 and 1969, an elevenfold increase in hemorrhoid operations and a sevenfold increase in operations for varicose veins had occurred.

And the prevalence of deep vein thrombosis and pulmonary embolism was also low in undeveloped communities in Africa, India, and Pakistan. Studies of autopsy reports showed that while these problems were discovered at death in 24 percent of United States whites and 22 percent of U.S. blacks, they were found in only 2 percent of Ugandan Africans.

In 110 of 114 mission hospitals in Africa checked by Burkitt, doctors estimated that they saw fewer than five cases of deep vein thrombosis yearly and more than half did not see one a year. And of 33 mission hospitals in India and Pakistan, 13 did not see one case and only five saw more than five cases. In a study at the Charles Johnson Memorial Hospital in Zululand, only three cases of thrombosis were discovered among 11,000 inpatients.

Before considering seriously that any one or all three of the vein conditions might relate, and if so how, to dietary changes, Burkitt had to consider the accepted ideas about causation.

He did take a hard look at those ideas—and, in the light of the epidemiological findings now, the evidence on the geographic distribution of all three diseases, the accepted ideas had to be found wanting.

Man's erect posture has usually been considered the most important causal factor in varicose veins because only human beings have the problem. Even as late as 1968, one of the best and most widely used British surgical textbooks, Bailey and Love's *Short Practice of Surgery,* dismissed the subject of etiology, or cause, with a single statement that varicose veins are part of the penalty we pay for the adoption of the upright posture. But that could hardly explain the fact that upright Africans rarely pay such a penalty.

A hereditary weakness in the vessel walls or valves has also been held to be a primary cause of varicose veins. But one strong argument against a primary influence of genetic endowment is the fact that varicose veins are now equally common in American blacks and whites, while the condition is still rare in parts of Africa from which American blacks came. Moreover, as one of Burkitt's reporting physicians noted, varicose veins are much more prevalent among New Zealand Maoris than among less Westernized but ethnically similar Polynesian islanders.

Another fact suggesting that heredity is not of primary causative importance in common diseases is that no true congenital deformity occurs in more than 0.5 percent of live births. As Cleave had pointed out, it is most unlikely that any disease such as varicosities more than twenty times as common as this could be primarily an inherited defect.

Burkitt also found evidence that in England deep vein thrombosis is less common among immigrants from India and Pakistan than in the indigenous population. In hospitals in Birmingham, England, in 1969, there were 138 cases among 46,500 patients who had been born in England, not one case among 1,976 born in India or Pakistan.

Burkitt's reporting physicians also confirmed the rarity of pulmonary embolism in Africans. Doctors from two hospitals in Nigeria and one in Zaire (formerly Belgian Congo), each admitting over 6,000 patients annually, could remember not one case of pulmonary embolism. Other physicians in Zaire and Kenya could remember only a single case each in more than twenty years' experience. From the King Edward Memorial Hospital in Bombay came a report that with 61,000 admissions annually, fatal pulmonary embolism was virtually unknown.

Prolonged standing is another commonly suggested cause. But there is no evidence that Africans or Indians stand for less time than Europeans or North Americans—and, in fact, many have identical or similar jobs, yet differ greatly in susceptibility to varicose veins.

Is pregnancy, as often alleged, a primary cause? That could hardly be since it was now clear that women in countries with low frequency of varicose veins have on average more pregnancies than those in communities with a high incidence.

And what of constrictive clothing? Again, that was hardly likely to play any significant role since women's dress in Western countries is no more constrictive than that worn by women in many countries where varicose veins are virtually unknown.

Hemorrhoids, too, have been attributed to man's erect posture, heredity, prolonged standing and, as late as 1963, one authority even included horseback riding.

Such proposed explanations could be offered—and were—on the basis of limited observation and experience by physicians familiar with the high incidence in European and North American patients. But they do not stand up once the differing incidence throughout the world is considered.

The long-accepted explanations have to be eliminated as being explanations of primary causes but, Burkitt believes, they could have some validity as contributory or aggravating factors in the presence of a primary cause.

Any adequate hypothesis to explain the cause of varicose veins, deep vein thrombosis, and hemorrhoids clearly would have to explain many observations and facts. Among them, certainly: the similarity in the geographical distribution of all three conditions; their rarity in all developing countries contrasted with their high incidence in more affluent communities; the striking contrast between the high incidence among American blacks and the low incidence in Africans; the company these diseases kept, the relation between them and other diseases such as diverticular disease, appendicitis, polyps, and cancer of the colon characteristic of economic development; and why the incidence of hemorrhoids in a community rises before that of varicose veins.

The only hypothesis that had been offered that could fulfill these needs was that of Cleave who had been arguing that the fundamental cause of these conditions is stool arrest that results from the fiber-depleted diet characteristic of Western civilization.

With that basic hypothesis of Cleave, Burkitt agreed entirely, even though he had to differ with Cleave on some of the mechanisms involved.

Cleave considered that it was local pressure exerted by the loaded bowel—constipated, full of slow-moving feces because of a fiber-depleted diet—that did the harm.

He believed that the loaded colon leaned on and exerted pressure in the abdomen on veins returning blood from the legs, interfering with normal blood flow, and thus causing veins in the legs to balloon out and become varicose. Similarly, Cleave saw the feces-loaded rectum exerting pressure there in veins in the rectal wall, causing them to balloon out and become hemorrhoidal. As for deep vein thrombosis, he again implicated pressure transmitted back to the leg veins because of the leaning of the loaded colon, and the leaning was all the greater when the patient was recumbent as after surgery. He claimed that the rapid rise in the incidence of deep vein thrombosis in the last twenty years could be related to the abandonment of the old routine hospital practice of emptying the colon by purgatives and enemas.

But Burkitt, as an experienced surgeon, could not accept the idea of a loaded colon leaning on veins in the abdomen. Nor could Neil Painter. "I promise you," says Painter, "that isn't true. Because I have deliberately felt for it at operation and there is no compression of a vein by the colon. That may happen in a cadaver in the anatomy room shriveled with Formalin but not in a living human being."

To Burkitt and Painter—and to many others now—there is a more valid mechanism. Painter had clearly established by now that a low fiber diet raises pressures within the colon, which result in diverticular disease. Moreover, constipation, resulting from a low fiber diet, not only raises pressures within the colon; it also necessitates straining at stool. And it had been demonstrated in several studies that straining at stool can raise pressures within the abdomen to as much as 200 milligrams of mercury.

Raised abdominal pressures are known to be readily transmittted to the superficial veins of the legs after the valves there have become defective. In fact, a physician testing for valve competence will ask a patient to cough since coughing raises abdominal pressures.

Valves, of course, are designed to help keep blood moving in one direction. They close behind the blood as it is pumped up from the legs to return to the heart. When they close, they are submitted to increases in abdominal pressure. And buffeted over an extended period of time by the high pressures induced by straining at stool, they may become less competent or effective in closing. Then the high pressures from straining at stool are freer to get through the valves and cause dilation and other changes in the leg veins.

When the outer, superficial veins of the leg become dilated, they become varicose veins. But the process does not necessarily stop there. As changes occur in the superficial visible veins, they are followed by changes in the veins connecting the superficial to the deep muscle veins. The latter then may undergo changes. And it seems probable to Burkitt that the changes in the deep muscle veins predispose them to cause blood to stagnate and clots to form when there is immobilization during serious illness or after surgery.

"This," he says, "could explain why deep vein thrombosis is so rare in developing countries where fiber intake is high and constipation and straining at stool are most uncommon—even in hospitals with operating conditions almost identical to those existing in Western countries.

"It has always been assumed in the Western world that deep vein thrombosis—and the aftermath of pulmonary embolism—is related to surgery or severe immobilizing illness. But if you go into hospitals in Delhi, Durban, or Kampala, you have the same operations, the same operating tables, the same anesthetics, the same catgut, the same instruments, and yet you have far less deep vein thrombosis."

Is he absolutely certain that it really is straining at stool which leads to all this?

No, not absolutely. "If," he says, "straining, as I believe, causes breakdown of valves and dilation of the superficial veins in the leg which you can see, it would be a very reasonable hypothesis that it might also cause changes in the deep veins which you don't see. The deep veins might stretch and become tortuous, and if there were such changes, then, during surgery and afterward with immobilization, with stagnation of blood flow, they would be more likely to clot than veins which are normal.

"We need to know more before we can be certain that changes—and what changes—do occur in the deep veins and we are doing studies now, a number of studies, to try to get definitive information.

"But certainly it is interesting that there are a number of hospitals in England—among them a big naval hospital, one of the best provincial hospitals, The Royal Berks in Reading, and a major Liverpool hospital—which have been feeding their patients high fiber diets, and all affirm that they have greatly reduced their prevalence of deep vein thrombosis."

Hemorrhoids, too, are related to raised abdominal pressures caused by straining at stool. And the observation that always, when traditional high fiber diet in a community gives way to more refined foods, the incidence of hemorrhoids rises before that of varicose veins can be explained by the fact that rectal veins, having no valves, are unprotected from abdominal pressures whereas the leg veins are initially protected by their valves.

Hiatus hernia is another characteristically Western disease. Cleave related it to diet but saw it as a matter of overconsumption of food. Burkitt ties it in with low fiber.

Hiatus hernia is a peculiar problem. It is now known to be one of the most prevalent defects in the gastrointestinal tract in the Western world. Hiatus comes from the Latin, *hiare,* to yawn, and a hernia is a rupture that permits an organ to protrude through it. In hiatus hernia (sometimes called hiatal hernia or sliding hernia), there is a defect in the diaphragm, the strong, dome-shaped muscle that separates the chest from the abdominal cavity. The esophagus, or gullet, passes through the diaphragm. And the defect is at the point in the diaphragm, just above the stomach, where the esophagus passes through.

Through this defect a part of the stomach may enter the chest cavity, either intermittently or constantly. Often, a hiatus hernia is symptomless but, not uncommonly, it is associated with esophageal reflux, an abnormal return flow of material, including gastric juices, from the stomach to the esophagus, and the reflux is a common cause of many troublesome upper abdominal symptoms.

With hiatus hernia and reflux, there may be heartburn, regurgitation, and burning pain in back of the breastbone, which is worse after eating and when lifting or stooping. Sometimes the pain may resemble the anginal chest pain associated with heart disease.

The diagnosis of hiatus hernia is made by X ray taken after a swallow of barium, a contrast material that helps to show up the defect. And the defect is often found in Western countries. In one U.S. study it showed up in one in five barium X-ray examinations. In a second U.S. study, a large one involving 2,402 examinations, it was found in 12.5 percent. In a study in England on patients not suspected of having hiatus hernia it was found in

29.6 percent of all the patients—in 21 percent of the males and 39 percent of the females—with the frequency rising with age, from 9 percent in those under forty to 69 percent in patients over seventy.

Yet, in studies he carried out with the aid of Dr. Peter A. James of Wythenshawe Hospital, Manchester, Burkitt found that hiatus hernia is rare in developing countries and almost unknown in communities that have departed little from their traditional way of life.

James himself, in seven years in Africa as the sole thoracic or chest surgeon in Uganda, had not seen a single case of hiatus hernia. On the other hand, James, back in England, in a series of just 200 barium X rays found 27 cases of significant hiatus hernia.*

In conversations and correspondence with many American surgeons and radiologists, Burkitt and James found none indicating any obvious disparity between the prevalence of hiatus hernia in white and black Americans. "Our hospital's population," Dr. Alvin Segel of Cuyahoga County Hospital, Cleveland, wrote them, "is approximately equally divided between white and black patients, and I do not believe there is any significant racial difference in the incidence of hiatus hernia."

Many explanations had been offered for hiatus hernia. When the upward protrusion of the stomach through the diaphragm was first recognized, it was believed to be a developmental abnormality, and the term "congenital short esophagus" was used to describe the condition. But later, because it was found to be relatively rare during the first three decades of life, it became recognized that it was an acquired, not congenital, defect.

Then, it seemed that the factors responsible for the stomach moving upward from its normal position below the diaphragm must be a push from below, a pull from above, a failure of the diaphragm to hold the junction between esophagus and stomach in the correct position, or a combination of these factors.

---

* And the data coming in to Burkitt from physicians in developing countries about the rarity of the condition in native populations was striking. In Nigeria not one case had been found in 800 X-ray examinations; in Kenya only 1 case in 1,319 examinations; in Tanzania one physician had found only one case in 733 examinations and a second had found only 2 in 1,206. Three different physicians in South Africa reported that the problem was "extremely uncommon." Reports from Calcutta indicated an incidence of less than 1 percent, and one study there found no case in 800 consecutive X-ray examinations. The incidence was less than 1 percent in Iraq, one per thousand examinations in Hong Kong, 14 minimal cases in 1,000 consecutive examinations in South Korea.

Some investigators blamed it on a contraction of the esophagus that pulled the stomach up, and they argued that the contraction was the result of ulceration produced by reflux or backward flow of the stomach contents. Others held that the stomach was pushed up because of increased pressures within the abdomen, and they attributed the pressure increases to such factors as tumors, pregnancy, obesity, and constrictive clothing. Still others held that the diaphragm weakened with age and let the stomach slip through.

But none of these arguments seemed at all convincing to Burkitt and James.

If the esophagus was contracted by reverse flow of stomach contents, what caused the reflux? The only explanation consistent with the geographical distribution of hiatus hernia was Cleave's. He argued that it was the availability of refined carbohydrate foods that encouraged people to eat too much—the refined, concentrated sweets and starches that went down so easily and led people to eat when they were not really hungry—that was responsible for abnormal gastric behavior and this predisposed to reflux.

Yet, that was difficult for Burkitt and James to accept. It seemed to them that any pathological changes in the esophagus are more likely to be the result of, rather than cause of, hiatus hernia.

As for the aging diaphragm, people in underdeveloped countries had aging diaphragms, too—but very little hiatus hernia.

Raised pressures within the abdomen pushing up the stomach? Yes, almost certainly, they are a major cause of hiatus hernia—but not, the two men agreed, raised pressures caused by factors to which they had been attributed.

Tumors as a cause of raised pressures? But abdominal tumors grow to much larger sizes in countries where surgical treatment is less readily available, and it is in just such countries that hiatus hernia is rare.

Pregnancy? But women have more rather than fewer pregnancies in countries where hiatus hernia is rare. And, as Cleave had remarked, it would be very strange if the human race had not adapted to such a normal condition as pregnancy.

Constrictive clothing? But if that were a causative factor, the incidence of hiatus hernia should have fallen rather than risen during the past twenty years.

Obesity? Obesity is often associated with hiatus hernia, but there is no evidence that it significantly raises abdominal pressures.

No, none of these but rather a fiber-depleted diet, Burkitt and James believe, can explain hiatus hernia.

Diverticular disease and hiatus hernia are closely associated epidemiologically. Their distribution appears to be almost identical: rare in developing countries, common in the developed. Available evidence suggests that both emerged as diseases of importance in Western countries at about the same time. They are both rare in people under thirty and their incidence increases strikingly with age. The many similarities suggest some causative factor they share in common.

And it is now clear that fiber-depleted diets are the major cause of constipation, and of the exaggerated contractions needed to propel through the bowel the small hard fecal content associated with low residue foods, and the contractions result in unnaturally raised pressures which, all the evidence indicates, are the fundamental cause of diverticular disease.

Not only is small hard fecal content responsible for raised pressures within the colon; it is the basic cause of straining at stool that raises pressures within the abdomen. They could well exert tremendous force upward and, after many years, push up the stomach, producing hiatus hernia.

Hiatus hernia, as already noted, is not always symptomatic. When it is severely so and nothing else helps, surgery may be used to repair the defect. But surgery is not commonly needed. Generally, patients with the problem have been advised to eat five or six small meals a day instead of three big ones, not to eat anything just before lying down, to keep the upper part of the chest elevated when lying down, to avoid stooping over, to elevate the head of the bed, to avoid wearing tight belts and other tight items of clothing. Antacids may be suggested to help neutralize stomach acids and cool off the burning esophagus. And with such measures symptoms have been relieved to a greater or lesser extent.

It would seem that resort to a high fiber diet might well speed the relief and perhaps promote healing of the defect by helping to eliminate the raised pressures. It might well, if used before hiatus hernia develops, prevent the development.

Peter Cleave would have another prescription. He would certainly not argue against a high fiber diet that he considers valuable for many other reasons. But he still argues earnestly that he cannot agree with Burkitt and James that hiatus hernia is related in any way to straining at stool. To him it is a matter of overconsumption. Hiatus hernia, he says, "stems in my opinion from the common practice in Westernized countries today of eating in the absence of hunger. I contend that any sufferer from heartburn and acid eructations will find that keeping the bowel open, whether by using unprocessed bran or otherwise, has no effect on these symptoms whatever, but that eating nothing for which he is not really hungry has an effect that is both striking and lasting."

10

A whole fresh view of obesity

A few years ago Dr. Hugh Trowell went back to East Africa on a visit and was astonished at the fat Africans. The towns were full of them and yet obesity had been very rare in East Africans in his time.

Trowell had first gone to Africa in 1929 and had spent almost thirty years there. As a young medical officer of the Kenya government, he had remarked that almost all Africans in Kenya in 1929 looked as thin as the ancient Egyptians. In six years in Kenya he had noticed that only an occasional chief could be considered "well covered." He had noticed, too, that when he was entertained in African homes, almost invariably, except in times of scarcity, food was left at the end of the meal and fed to domestic pets.

During World War II, he was aware, a team of British medical experts had been formed and sent to Africa to advise the military authorities about army diets because Africans refused to eat the number of calories that nutritionists, including Trowell himself, advised.

"Hundreds of X rays," he recalls, "were taken of African intestines in an effort to solve the mystery that lay in the fact that everyone knew how to fatten a chicken for the pot, but no one knew how to make Africans eat their calorie requirements and put on flesh and fat for battle. It remained an unsolved mystery."

And yet now there was the amazing spectacle of towns full of fat Africans.

Hugh Trowell, a most distinguished physician, awarded the

Order of the British Empire for his remarkable work elucidating the nature of the disease kwashiorkor,* was back in Africa at the invitation of the Uganda government. A special commemorative meeting was being held at the Makerere medical school in honor of the late Sir Albert Cook, who had been a great and famed medical missionary in Uganda. Trowell had been consultant physician at Makerere; he had also been personal physician to Sir Albert; he was there to give a talk about the work of Sir Albert.

And it was there that he met Denis Burkitt again and heard Burkitt talk at the meeting on the hypothesis that many diseases of the Western world were associated with refined carbohydrates and a fiber-deficient diet—and, with good personal reason, Trowell was struck by the concept and, coming out of medical retirement, almost immediately began to make important contributions to it, relating it to obesity and then to diabetes and coronary heart disease as well.

Hugh Trowell had known Denis Burkitt and known him well. It was Trowell, as we have seen, who had shown Burkitt his first case of Burkitt's lymphoma, although it was not, of course, called that then.

Trowell had left Kampala in 1958 to return home to England because of the ill health of his wife, Margaret, a remarkable woman in her own right, who had become interested in the potential of Africans for art and had given art lessons on the back veranda of her home, established an art school, and whose work had so influenced the burgeoning and appreciation of native art that, when she went home, the art school in Makerere College was given her name—the Margaret Trowell School of Fine Art.

Trowell's kwashiorkor work had been full of difficulties, even extraordinary difficulties. For years he had had to fight not only

* Kwashiorkor, which means "the sickness that the older child gets when the next baby is born," has been called by the World Health Organization "the most widespread and severe nutritional disorder known to medical science." But it was not recognized as a nutritional disease until the work of Trowell and another government physician, Cicely Williams. It produced children with fleshless skulls and bloated abdomens, and it could kill and often did. It was a mystery to physicians except to some who dismissed it as being a manifestation of congenital syphilis. Some, along with African mothers, regarded it as the "weaning disease," although they had no clear idea of what it involved. Some thought it was pellagra, a vitamin deficiency disease. It was the work of Hugh Trowell and Cicely Williams—and Trowell's book on the disease in 1952—that established that kwashiorkor was the result of protein deficiency and where nothing else had been effective protein feeding was lifesaving.

to gain acceptance for the idea that kwashiorkor was a nutritional disease caused by protein deficiency; even to get consideration for that possibility and support for trying to treat the disease with protein had been difficult. He had even been contacted by Communist agents who sought to persuade him to say that kwashiorkor in Africa was due to capitalistic colonialism even though the disease had been occurring for centuries.

Upon arriving in England, he retired from medicine, took holy orders, and became the Reverend Dr. Hugh Carey Trowell, vicar of Stratford-sub-Castle in Salisbury.

Even as he entered the ministry Trowell did undertake to complete one project carried over from his experiences in Africa—a book called *Noninfective Diseases in Africa*, which was published in 1960.

In it he noted that many noninfective diseases common in Westernized countries were rare in Africa. They were many of the same diseases that Cleave had listed, particularly those of the bowel: constipation, appendicitis, diverticular disease, hemorrhoids, ulcerative colitis, irritable colon, polyps, and cancer of the colon and rectum.

It was a very careful, precise, well-documented, highly scientific volume. It sold only a handful of copies. In it Trowell did not advance seriously any hypothesis or theory as to why such diseases were rare among Africans. But he did make a few significant observations.

"The natural African diets," he wrote, "are usually high in their fiber content, which is often more than 15 percent, and manual workers must consume a bulky diet to satisfy their caloric requirements. There is therefore a bulky residue left in the abdomen, and the next large meal sets up a marked gastrocolic reflex and desire to evacuate. True constipation is uncommon in Africans.

"In towns and under the modern way of life, refined flours, sugar, fats, and other foods form a large part of the diet, which may contain little fiber, few vegetables and fruit. Less food also is consumed for the caloric requirements of the sedentary worker are less. Numerous small meals of purified foods and a tense, worried manner of life all conspire to upset normal defecation reflexes. The fecal mass passes sluggishly along the colon and is evacuated as small, desiccated, fecal masses rather than the bulky, soft, pultaceous stool of the peasant engaged in manual toil.

"While it would be fanciful to ascribe the pattern of colonic diseases in Africa entirely to a combination of the soft bulky stool and a placid temperament, yet it is an interesting idea and indeed a generalization to which there are many exceptions."

It was hardly any wonder that Hugh Trowell was fascinated when he heard Denis Burkitt talk that day at Makerere.

It was not that he wanted to leave the ministry. And he has not even as of now, still carrying on some of the duties of a churchman in his spare time—and he makes time for them. But he knew that day that he had to get back into medical research and he has been back ever since.

Obesity was one research project for him.

Many Africans—in the towns—had changed markedly even within ten years. Could their obesity now have anything to do with a dietary change? Could obesity elsewhere, around the world, wherever it was a major problem, have anything to do or much to do with such a dietary change? If obesity had become a problem only recently in Africa, when, in fact, had it become a problem elsewhere?

Curiously, although hundreds upon hundreds of medical and popular books, and medical and popular articles have been written on the subject of obesity, Trowell could find no reference in any of them to the history of the disorder.

There is a popular current theory that man has an appetite center in the hypothalamus of the brain—a kind of "stat" control center somewhat akin to a thermostat. And the theory holds that somehow this center has to break down for obesity to occur.

If little has been known about the history of obesity—about when it became a widespread severe problem—Trowell, a small, gentle, patient, and lovingly scholarly man, could look long and hard into it. And he could produce evidence—from the English language and literature and from the art of many countries—that widespread severe obesity is a modern phenomenon, and if there is an appetite center, then its breakdown must be peculiarly a modern phenomenon, occurring in Western man only during the last three centuries and only now in developing countries.

Logically enough, Trowell consulted the *Oxford English Dictionary*. It is emphatic that the word obese was rarely used before the nineteenth century. Nor had alternative terms—stout, corpulent, or even fat—been in common use before the nineteenth century. Yet, there was no lack of words to describe thinness and leanness, and many descriptions of this condition go back to antiquity and are to be found in all ancient literature.

Trowell found that the word obese was first used for animals artificially fed up for slaughter, and when it was first applied to humans it did not mean obese but rather well fed, plump. The word, in fact, comes from the Latin *obesus,* meaning "having eaten" and not signifying fatness. Searching the classical literature of Rome and Greece, Trowell could find no clear description of a historical person who was obese. But there were *obesi*—statues of thin elderly Roman men reclining on couches, their abdomens bulging after a feast.

The outstanding feature of almost all statues, wall paintings, tomb and temple reliefs of ancient Assyria, Egypt, Greece, and Rome, Trowell found, is that men and women were regularly depicted as thin in body and limb. The classical Venus of Praxiteles of the fourth century B.C. and the Venus of Milo of a later century both depicted the ideal feminine form rounded in contours but with no suspicion of excessive fat.

Shakespeare did not use the term obese and resorted to the term fat only on rare occasions, such as the "old fat woman" in the *Merry Wives of Windsor*. Falstaff was Shakespeare's only man of any girth, "a good portly man of faith and corpulence."

"Anyone," Hugh Trowell will tell you, "who wishes to know when obesity appeared in the English upper classes might walk about the National Portrait Gallery in Trafalgar Square in London where are to be found portraits of all the monarchs from the fourteenth century on. But no obesity at all is to be seen in royalty or statesmen until Henry VIII had a slight double chin toward the end of the fifteenth century. Charles II in the second half of the seventeenth century is the first monarch with a pronounced paunch, a really obese abdomen. Toward the end of the seventeenth century every noble man and noble lady is depicted, quite suddenly, as invariably obese."

What was happening?

Obesity in the English upper classes at that time and in the eighteenth century could be attributed to the dawning age of elegance. Many technological changes were occurring in basic industries. The agricultural revolution was beginning to provide much more food, at least for the upper classes. Meat, milk, and butter increased, and sugar imported from the recently founded West Indies colonies began to be used in coffee, chocolate, and tea, and then in cakes and puddings.

It was also then that a new grinding system of milling provided flours of different qualities. In all, some of the bran was sifted out.

But the grades that contained the least bran were much prized by the upper classes even though they were more expensive. The palest flour, with the least bran, became a status symbol and was desired by the lower classes in England. But among the latter the change from high fiber flour to low fiber flour and thus from whole-meal bread to white bread took place slowly and irregularly during the eighteenth and nineteenth centuries.

There must surely, Trowell could think, be some connection between the changes in the feeding habits of the upper classes in England in the eighteenth century—and in others of the most sophisticated Western nations—and the appearance of gross obesity among the gentry in all those nations.

And there must, he reasoned, be the same connection between the growing incidence of obesity among Africans in recent years and the changes in feeding habits among them.

And Trowell, carrying on his obesity research with the aid of a grant from the British Heart Association, could soon begin to formulate a hypothesis about appetite control and what the change in feeding habits did to it.

Not only did primates consume starch—always with much fiber in shoots, leaves, and fruit—and remain thin; so had primitive man, the hunter, who, often unable to satisfy his hunger on game, continued to eat starch and fiber in shoots, berries, and fruit, his appetite center geared to this diet. Obesity would have been a heavy liability to hunter (or hunted) and subsequently to man, the cereal eater, who grew his own crops, and still took most of his food as carbohydrate with its full complement of fiber. Obesity did not occur in primitive man who adapted well to cereals.

Modern physical activity often requires a diet providing only 2,000 to 2,500 calories a day, 1,000 calories less than for primitive man. Fats and proteins, both without fiber, have increased in the modern diet. And carbohydrates, which provide about 50 percent of the calories, now also contain little cereal dietary fiber.

Significantly, out of a typical modern diet, 93.2 percent of the available energy in the foods could be absorbed. That is high. Many research studies showed that if the diet was altered to contain brown bread, fruit, and vegetables, the figure went down to 91.1 percent. And on whole-meal bread, it was cut further to 88–89 percent; there was decreased digestion and absorption of food in diets that are rich in fiber.

"That latter figure, 88–89%," says Trowell, "is, I suggest, the figure that is the natural, inherited, evolutionary figure" to keep body weight at a natural level.

Africans on high fiber diets, Trowell points out, not only have colons twice the size of modern Western man, and stool weight double and transit time three times as rapid, and a low incidence of certain diseases of the colon; they have all this together with full stomachs after meals on bulky fiber-rich carbohydrates, which are digested and absorbed more slowly, allowing satiety mechanisms to operate normally to preserve normal weight throughout life, even when physical activity decreases during middle age.

Like Western man, when they switch to westernized low fiber diets, they lose their natural protection from obesity.

Cleave, too, argued that it was time for a whole new look at the problem of obesity. That, certainly, it was not primarily the result of a fault in the instinct of appetite—"such as the mysterious derangement, postulated by some, of a hypothetical 'appestat' center in the brain." And that, too, the primary cause was not any dislike of and abstention from taking exercise.

"No wild creature is ever overweight," Cleave insisted. "The forces of evolution have ensured that in nature organisms react to an abundant food supply never by developing a disease such as obesity." As long as any organism, including man, lives under natural conditions, there is no obesity.

Exercise? Throughout the whole animal kingdom, no living creature, unless forced to do so in order to get food, ever takes any more exercise than it wants to take.

And even when animals are confined, as in zoos, so that lack of exercise is imposed on them, obesity does not occur unless food is tampered with. In a zoo, Cleave says, you see "the two opposite poles of creation—a large animal like a tiger, accustomed to hunt its prey over many square miles of jungle, and now confined to a space measured in cubic feet; and a small bird, like a finch, accustomed to fly about many acres of countryside, and now confined to a space measured in cubic inches. In each case the natural exercise has been enormously reduced. Yet, just because each of these creatures continues to take its food in its natural form, in the one case raw meat and bones, and in the other case unaltered seeds, the weight remains the same and obesity does not occur."

As forcefully as he can say it, Peter Cleave has long said and continues to say: "The *sole* (and this is his emphasis) cause of obesity lies in the consumption of refined carbohydrates. A large appetite is not a cause, and a dislike of exercise is not a cause."

It is true, Cleave agrees, that restraining the appetite or enforcing exercise will reduce obesity, "but as long as the true cause continues to operate—the consumption of refined carbohydrates—the use of either is an example of two wrongs not making a right. To be sure, these two factors are valuable in the removal of surplus weight already in existence, but in the basic matter of prevention the mind should be riveted on the essential cause and not confused by irrelevancies."

The Cleave argument and the Trowell hypothesis were not only to be reinforced but amplified considerably and graphically by a brilliant young gastroenterologist, Dr. Kenneth W. Heaton, consultant, senior lecturer in medicine at the Universty of Bristol Department of Medicine, Bristol Royal Infirmary in England.

Until 1969 Heaton's major research interest had certainly not been obesity. He had some interest in it as a physician because it was a very common problem among patients he saw. But his major research interest was bile, bile salts, bile salt metabolism, and gallstones, about which he is now considered one of the world's foremost authorities—and, in fact, his work in this area very much enters into this story, too, as we shall see at a later point.

In 1969 Heaton had not been back long from a year as a research fellow at Duke University in the States, working in the bile salt area, when he happened to pick up some writings of Peter Cleave.

He was impressed. It seemed to him that Cleave's concept of the role of refined carbohydrates not only in obesity but in other diseases had much to be said for it. He was impressed enough to take to it personally.

When I visited Ken Heaton in his office at the Bristol Royal Infirmary, I asked him to tell me all that happened and he did it so cogently and concisely that I will let him tell it here again.

"I took Cleave's arguments seriously enough in 1969 to change my diet, excluding sugar as completely as I could, and white flour as completely as I could, and all refined carbohydrates, too. I did it on general health grounds, not because I was obese. I wasn't overweight at all. But I lost weight—much to my surprise. I am down fifteen pounds from what I was when I made the change.

My weight now is less than it was when I left Cambridge at twenty-one. I am 6′3″ and I weigh 147 pounds, and that is thin and I admit it. But I am extremely healthy and I have never been healthier than in these last five years. In terms of trivial infections and the like, I have never had fewer.

"And my whole family is the same because we are all on the same diet. My wife, who is a physician, also lost about ten pounds, unexpectedly.

"We don't have any restrictions on caloric intake at all. We eat as much as we want. We don't normally use bran—but we do use whole-meal bread and avoid artificially sweetened foods. That's all. We use perhaps a teaspoonful of sugar a day in our family diet. I must have a bit of marmalade at breakfast but otherwise I practically have no sugar at all.

"I have a colleague here who joined us in 1971 and he was sufficiently impressed, too, for him and his family to go on this diet. And they also involuntarily lost weight. He lost two stone—twenty-eight pounds; his wife, a stone or more.

"The crux, I think, is this: what is it about removing fiber from the diet which makes food fattening, to use simple language? Cleave, you know, says refining concentrates food, and that's the problem. I was attracted to that idea but was never entirely happy about it.

"And then it occurred to me—I had to give a talk, in fact, to some dietitians—that what actually happens when you remove fiber is that you change the physical state of the food, which changes the demands that the food makes upon your digestive tract.

"You know, extracting nutrients from fiber-rich foods is precisely what our digestive tracts are designed for. And they are seemingly efficient at doing this. If you process the foods in such a way that they are already extracted, the fiber removed, you have usurped the function of the digestive tract and taken away from it something it is perfectly capable of doing, and you are asking it to process food which has already been processed.

"Now this is an idea which needs a great deal more working out, but it seems to me logical that we may well disturb the functioning of the GI tract if we ask it to act upon foods that have already been acted upon.

"Perhaps this is a bit woolly so far, but if we look at the very first part of your body to touch food, your teeth, what are the teeth there for, what have they been evolved for? To chew food, of course. To cope with food which requires chewing, which is in a physical state such that it must be broken up in order to extract nutrients from it.

"And what is it that makes food have properties that require chewing? In plant food, it is fiber. Fiber is the skeleton which gives strength and cohesion to the plant, and it is because plants have this strength and cohesion that animals have to break them up, grind them with their teeth, in order to get nutrients out of them.

"So the very fact that we have teeth proves that we are adapted to fiber.

"It has sometimes been suggested that we were originally carnivores. But I don't think that's valid. Because we are supposedly descended from the trees, and our ancient ancestors would be fruit-eating, apelike animals. When man's ancestors took to the ground and started hunting, they didn't hunt as lions and other carnivores hunt. They hunted with bows and arrows and stones and used implements rather than bare hands and bare teeth to get the meat off. I think basically man has fruit-eating teeth; human dentition is nearest to a fruit-eating animal's rather than to a carnivore's.

"So, we have teeth to chew, and one of the properties of fiber is that it demands to be chewed. You cannot eat fiber-rich food without chewing. But the minute you remove the fiber, you produce a food which no longer requires to be chewed.

"In the case of sugar, when you extract it from the beet or the cane, you produce a material you can actually drink, whereas if you wanted to get the sugar from the original cane or beet, you would have had to chew like hell. And if you want to get sugar from a normal source—fruit—you have to chew. So that with our sugar refineries we have turned sugar from a material which in nature always had to be chewed into a material which can be ingested with no chewing whatever.

"In removing, we change the physical state. We do it with sugar and we do it with refined white flour. In an experiment done twenty years ago, it was shown that volunteers who took 45 minutes to eat a loaf of whole-meal bread took only 32 minutes to eat an equivalent white loaf—simply because the whole-meal loaf took more chewing.

"So the fact that refined foods need so much less chewing or none at all, making them so much easier and quicker to ingest, is one critical fact about the role of fiber.

"But, other than that, food which lacks fiber has had removed from it some nonnutritive material. When you eat a fiber-containing food, part of it is nonnutritive; it isn't absorbed; it doesn't supply calories. You get less energy than if you eat the same amount of fiber-depleted food.

"So a second property of fiber is that it has a space-filling effect. And that acts as an obstacle to energy intake, too. The first obstacle is that fiber must be chewed and that slows down ingestion; the second obstacle is that fiber displaces nutrients.

"And the third obstacle is that fiber promotes satiety. Now this is theoretical at the moment but I think it fits all the facts. If you chew a food, it is more satisfying. The reason is that the act of chewing stimulates the secretion of saliva and also the secretion of gastric juices. And both the saliva and the juices are there in the stomach, along with the food, helping to fill the stomach and promote satiety. But if you eat fiber-depleted food, requiring little or no chewing, producing far less juices, the stomach is less distended and you feel less full or satisfied.

"So in three different ways fiber acts as an obstacle to energy intake and to obesity.

"I know that other reasons for obesity are commonly advanced. I am very unimpressed by the idea that lack of exercise causes obesity, just as Cleave is. I know of no experimental evidence—no experiment—in which a group of people who are normally pretty active have been made to restrain their activities and have been maintained on the same diet and have gained weight. It may exist but I don't know of it.

"If people have an instinct in them to take exercise, they can take it—go for a walk, a run, a cycle ride, or whatever they want to do. There are more swimming pools, tennis courts, squash courts, golf courses, and the like available than ever before in history. If people don't use them, it is because they don't want to use them. And if they don't want to use them, it may be that they don't need to use them.

"You get yourself into a situation—if you believe in the lack of exercise theory—of having to believe that man kept his weight down in primitive times because the stringent demands of agriculture before laborsaving devices came in forced him to exercise. But in primitive communities today people don't all take large amounts of exercise. I get the impression that the average African villager likes to lie under the banana tree as much as he can—and he isn't obese.

"I think we are obsessed with exercise as a means of combating obesity. But no practical evidence exists that it is necessary. It is extraordinary how much acceptance the importance of exercise for obesity has had without any real evidence. It is, I think, a kind of moral reaction to feelings of guilt about not working as hard as our ancestors.

"I suspect that if you looked for a correlation between the prevalence of obesity and the number of sports stadia and other artificial facilities for taking exercise, you would probably find that they go hand in hand: where people are obese there are more of these facilities.

"And there are theories about obesity, other than the lack of exercise one, that seem to boil down to mysterious, almost mystical, things going wrong in the hypothalamus or in the brain somewhere. This is obviously rubbish because man presumably is as highly evolved and adapted to his environment as any other animal species, and no other species gets obesity, except in one or two special cases before hibernating and that is natural, physiological, not pathological.

"Obesity is purely a human disease. That is absolutely a fact.

"They say people overeat because there is such a plentitude of food around. But, as Cleave says, no animal ever eats too much even with plenty available. Animals just don't overeat because they are eating their natural foods; they eat until satisfied; and what they eat is not only the right amount to satisfy them but the right amount so far as energy intake is concerned.

"I believe with Cleave that if man restricted himself to unprocessed foods, he would not suffer obesity except in rare and special circumstances. He is obese because the foods he eats are artificially easy to ingest and unsatisfying. He is not overeating. He is eating foods with an artificially high energy to satiety ratio. It's not his appetite center that's at fault and producing an abnormal demand for satiety. It's the foods that are at fault because they've been changed so that an abnormally large amount is needed for normal satiety.

"I can usually convince a lay person of the sense of this. But I get the feeling when I talk to medical audiences that they are very suspicious of this line of argument. And I think it is because it is an argument and I am not producing a series of experimental results, statistics, etc., because it is an argument which requires them to use their own intelligence and common sense and logical reasoning.

"I am being very rude about some members of my profession.

I am sorry but even the other day when I gave a lecture to a very distinguished audience, including several professors, I was taken up on this very point. They said, your arguments sound reasonable, but what is the evidence? And I replied, for goodness sake, use the evidence of your own common sense.

"I often use a slide. It shows a can of Coke which contains, I suspect to your surprise and certainly to most people's, 38 grams of sucrose, which is the equivalent of 10 sugar lumps, or 4½ to 5 teaspoonfuls of sugar. One single 11½-fluid-ounce can has that.

"And next to the can are four eating apples, medium size, just under one pound. They also contain 38 grams of sugar. So you have an example of refined sugar and an example of unrefined—two ways of getting 38 grams of sugar.

"And I simply ask, which of those will be easiest and quickest to take, and which will satisfy you most? Isn't the answer obvious? Do you need an experiment? Anyone who has eaten one apple knows that to eat four would leave you feeling stuffed, whereas with a can of Coke you can just quench your thirst and go on half an hour later to have a meal.

"I have thought long and hard about setting up an experiment in which a large number of people eating an ordinary diet containing refined carbohydrates swap it for an unrefined diet. I think most people would lose weight when sugar, white flour, and white rice are excluded. I have drawn up protocols for such an experiment and even started one but have fallen foul of practical difficulties in getting a large number of people to change diet and following them to make certain.

"The experiment, I suppose, must be done. But one of the tantalizing things is that similar experiments have been done before and produced evidence which would support the case.

"In a study in Cape Town, fifty-one male office workers were instructed to cut out sugar-containing foods but to try and maintain their weight by eating more of other foods. They failed to maintain their weight. After five months, their weight was on average three pounds less than when they started. Some men involuntarily lost more than five pounds.

"Similarly, in San Francisco, thirteen men already on a cholesterol-lowering diet were instructed to reduce the carbohydrate content of the diet by cutting out all sugar. Although the altered diet was designed so that it provided the same number of calories as the original cholesterol-lowering one, the men's weight fell by an average of four pounds in six months.

"In both of these, it was only sugar that was excluded, not other refined carbohydrates. It's likely that if others were excluded, there would have been greater weight loss."

Not long ago, Ken Heaton gave a lecture to a meeting of the British Dietetic Association in which he noted another significant experiment. In it ten young women were fed three diets of differing fiber content. Diet 1 contained white bread and no fruit or vegetables except potatoes—a low residue diet. Diet 2 contained whole-meal bread and some fruit and vegetables, while diet 3 contained more of these unrefined full-fiber foods and could be called a high fiber diet.

As the amount of fiber in the diet went up, so did the excretion of energy, of fat, and of nitrogen. Or, looking at it the other way, the less residue the diet had, the more energy these young women got out of their food. Energy in food is available only to the extent that it is absorbed by the intestine. Energy excreted in the stool is energy not available to the body. And the careful experiment demonstrated clearly that raising the intake of dietary fiber raises the excretion of energy in the stool.

Important for combating obesity?

"I should like to suggest," said Heaton, "that overnutrition is not normally due to overeating, to eating too much food. It is due to *getting too much out of food.* It is due to satisfying a normal appetite with food which has an artificially high energy/satiety ratio. In practice, this means refined carbohydrate.

"If this concept of how overnutrition arises is correct, then it follows that carbohydrate is only fattening when it is refined. Unrefined carbohydrate foods should be nonfattening, since their energy/satiety ratio has not been tampered with. Bread should be nonfattening if it is whole meal. (It is hard to believe that grass seeds, that is, wheat grains, are fattening!) Whole-meal flour contains 9 percent fewer calories per gram than white flour and it is 4 percent less absorbed. May I, therefore, make a plea to include whole-meal bread routinely in weight-reducing diets?"

11

The trail of some stones and some very key salts

GALLBLADDERS can be troublesome. Some animal species have them, some do not; and, confusingly, it can go either way in some species; some giraffes have them and some do not. Commonly, "nervy" people, those with considerable effrontery or "chutzpah," are said to have "plenty of gall." But we all do, in fact.

Gall—actually, bile salts—is produced by the liver and flows to the gallbladder, which is a kind of "side pocket," a temporary holding place. A pear-shaped sac, it holds an ounce or two. And when foods, especially fatty foods, leave the stomach and enter the duodenum, the first part of the small intestine, a signal goes to the gallbladder, which then promptly releases some gall that very neatly emulsifies or breaks up the fats so they can be absorbed.

But gallbladders can be troublesome—or, to put it more accurately, the cholesterol in gall can be. Cholesterol, blamed as it often is for being hazardous to the heart, sometimes can have another hazard, precipitating out of the gall to make small crystals that grow into gallstones.

Sometimes? Much too many times. Almost entirely because of gallstones, one-third of a million gallbladders are removed each year in the United States. In American women gallbladder removal—cholecystectomy—is a more common operation than appendectomy. American Indians have the highest known prevalence of gallstones of any population, with Indian women developing the disease at a remarkably early age.

In England, where cholecystectomy is the commonest elective

abdominal operation, over 40 percent of women and 20 percent of men are destined to develop gallstones by their seventies. In Sweden the odds are even higher, and in other European countries it appears that the situation is much the same, as it is in Australia.

Gallstones are not always symptomatic but when they are they can be agonizingly so. The victim may feel pain in the upper right abdomen and the pain may radiate to chest or back. There may be chills and fever, gas, heartburn, nausea, and vomiting. If the gallbladder should contract to try to expel an obstructing stone, there may be colic pains severe enough to take the breath away.

A mysterious condition? So gallstone formation has been for a long time. But now epidemiological studies—of where the condition occurs and where it does not—have provided valuable clues.

And some very remarkable and intricate detective work—a good deal of which has been done by Ken Heaton and his colleagues at Bristol—recently has been showing what apparently is specifically involved in gallstone formation and providing indications of how it may be prevented.

And, of course, you will have surmised that our old friends, refined carbohydrates, are involved. They are—and the discovery of how they are, if you like the picking apart of a puzzle and the putting together of bits of evidence to provide a clarifying picture, is a fascinating story.

Is gallstone formation a universal phenomenon?

Published reports on gallstone frequency in developing countries have been relatively few. In itself, this suggests that the disease is not common since absence of a problem naturally provokes less comment than its presence.

What reports have been published do indicate that gallstones are a rarity in sub-Saharal Africa. In Ghana a study of 4,395 autopsies showed not a single case. At Ibadan University Hospital over a 5-year period, only 27 patients with the disease were admitted and those tended to be wealthy, obese, and consumers of a westernized diet.

Burkitt, in his years of surgical practice in East Africa, operated on only two patients with gallstones—one of whom was a queen. And reports to Burkitt from mission hospitals indicated rarity.*

---

* In Uganda 12 hospitals supplying a total of 109 monthly returns thus far have not reported a single case of gallstones. The same is true of Malawi after 102

Of theories about what might possibly cause gallstone formation, there has hardly been any shortage.

One, for example, held that the stones are formed because of biliary stasis, or stoppage of bile flow, which, in turn, was the result of sedentary existence or tight corsets. For years no credence has been given to it.

For a hundred years infection of the gallbladder has been a popular explanation for stone formation but has been discounted for lack of any evidence.

More recently, diet has received consideration. Civilized diets contain refined carbohydrates but they also contain saturated animal fat. And such fat has been indicted. Yet, animal foods are expensive and refined carbohydrate is cheap, and in today's affluent societies it is not just the rich who get gallstones; the poor have the highest risk. The deprived Indian is the American who gets most gallstones and in Britain it is the relatively poor Northerner. In past centuries, when refined carbohydrate was expensive, it was the richer social classes who were most prone to gallstone formation. At one point, not too long ago, there was an idea that, all told, the fats in our diet were too much of the saturated kind and the trouble might be a deficiency of the polyunsaturated kind. But then in 1973 that idea was knocked out by the discovery that volunteers eating a diet rich in polyunsaturated fatty acids actually had an even higher incidence of gallstones.

Refined carbohydrate? Beyond those already mentioned above, there were other reasons why, conceivably, refined carbohydrate might be involved in gallstone formation.

---

hospital-months. In Tanzania only two cases have been reported in 207 hospital-months; in Kenya one case in 67 hospital-months; and in West Africa 13 Nigerian hospitals have seen only two gallstone patients in a total of 109 months.

And, following the same familiar pattern of other diseases common in Westernized countries and uncommon in developing countries, especially among natives staying with old ways of living and eating, the gallstone incidence, too, increases in the developing countries with the degree of urbanization and westernization. Africans in cities of Africa seem far more prone to gallstones than rural Africans. In autopsy studies in Johannesburg stones have been found in 10 percent of Bantu women in their forties. In Accra, where gallstones were unknown twenty years ago, they recently have been accounting for 0.4 percent of surgical admissions to hospitals.

Notably, too, since the Canadian Eskimo, rarely a sufferer from gallstones while living in his traditional nomadic way, has taken to living in towns like Inuvik, where Western practices are popular, gallstones have become so common that a 1971 report found cholecystectomies outnumbering all other surgical procedures.

There is the association of refined carbohydrate with obesity—and the association of obesity, in turn, with gallstones has long been recognized. Some studies have shown gallstone patients weighing on the average twelve pounds more than others without gallstones. Since World War II, gallstones have been increasing in men and in the young, paralleling an increase in obesity in men and in the young.

Diabetics have increased proneness to gallstones, and patients with gallstones are diabetic twice as often as expected. And Pima Indians in Arizona, who are usually obese, have the world's highest prevalence of diabetes and gallstones. It has long been well known that obesity and diabetes often go together—in fact, commonly do—in the same patient. It would seem that the three problems—obesity, gallstones, and diabetes—could share a causative factor in common. And, as we will see in a later chapter, there is increasing evidence now for an important role for refined carbohydrate in diabetes.

Significantly, too, animals, if they are given artificial diets, can be made to develop gallstones. Seven different groups of researchers have achieved gallstone formation in young hamsters, rabbits, and other animals, all with diets highly artificial and abnormal for any animal. Superficially, they look like very varied and different diets even if abnormal. Yet, they all have one thing in common: the carbohydrate in them is always refined, fiber-depleted carbohydrate so that none of the diets contains significant amounts of dietary fiber.

But exactly how does fiber work to reduce the likelihood of gallstone formation and its absence encourage it?

Therein lies the story of some ingenious experiments with humans and some remarkable putting of pieces of evidence together.

To follow what went on you need to know a few basic facts about bile salts and what happens to them.

The liver produces two bile salts that go into the bile. One is cholate; the second is chenodeoxycholate; and for brevity and simplicity we will refer to them here as C and CD respectively. They are called primary bile salts because they are made by the liver and circulate as such. They go, in the bile, to the gallbladder and, from there, when needed, they flow through a duct into the duodenum, the first part of the small intestine.

In the duodenum they go to work on fatty materials, breaking them up for digestion and absorption. And, having done that job by the time the fatty materials have moved along lower in the small intestine, the two salts, to a large extent, are reabsorbed and go by a special enterohepatic (intestinal/liver) circulatory system back to the liver for reuse.

But some of the two salts do move on in the intestinal tract and get into the large intestine, or colon. And there they are attacked by bacteria present in the colon. The bacteria turn the C salt (cholate) into a third salt, deoxycholate, which we will refer to here as D. D is reabsorbed in the colon and eventually it returns to the liver, which looks upon it kindly and reuses D for further outpouring of bile as if D were really unchanged C.

So we have a kind of recirculating bile salt pool—made up of the primary salts C and CD and the secondary salt D.

What effect did dietary fiber have on this whole business? Dr. Heaton and a colleague in Bristol, Dr. E. W. Pomare, a research fellow, decided to try to see what happened by feeding dietary fiber in the form of bran.

Healthy women were volunteer subjects. They were given an injection of tagged—radioactively labeled—C salt. And on each of the next four mornings, through a tube carefully inserted downward through the throat, esophagus, and stomach to the duodenum, a sample of bile was sucked up from the duodenum. By analyzing the bile sample, Heaton and Pomare could determine how much of the tagged C salt had been changed to the D salt. And, as expected, from morning to morning, there was a steady increase in the D salt in the bile, reflecting the fact that some of the tagged C was going to the colon, being acted on there by bacteria and changed to D, and the D was being reabsorbed in the colon, getting to the liver, and being circulated from the liver again in the bile pool.

Then, the very patient women were given bran as a supplement to their normal diet, taking about 33 grams (about four heaping teaspoonfuls) a day in divided doses with their meals, over a period of six to ten weeks. And at that point bile samples were again taken after injection of tagged C.

Now there was very definitely less D salt in the bile. The proportion of it in the bile fell by about half.

Did that mean that more of the C salt was being absorbed in the small intestine and less was reaching the colon to be acted upon by bacteria and converted to the D salt? That was highly improbable. If anything, the bran effect would be to carry more of C into the colon, to sweep it along.

That meant, then, that either less D was formed in the colon or less was absorbed from the colon. But if it was a case of less being absorbed, then there should be more excreted in the stool.

But more was not excreted in the stool. At the University of Edinburgh, Dr. Martin Eastwood, studying the amount of bile salts in the feces, found that there was as much of the D salt in the stools of subjects taking bran as in those not taking it. And other studies reported in 1971 had shown that in Afro-Asian communities, where a high fiber diet is eaten, the feces contain less, not more, D salt than in Western society.

The data, therefore, suggested that dietary fiber reduces the formation of the D salt.

"Now this, we thought," says Ken Heaton, "was interesting enough to report—and we did report it in the British *Medical Journal* late in 1973—because it shows that bran alters what is going on in the colon, altering colon physiology over and above increasing stool bulk and speeding transit time. It actually alters a metabolic function of the colon."

Still, Heaton did not have much of a clue at the time to what the significance of the reduced formation of the D salt might be.

"But, then," he says, "by extraordinary coincidence it happened that one of my colleagues here, Tom Low-Beer, developed an hypothesis that the D salt has a special role in the bile salt picture."

That role, Low-Beer thought, was to act as an inhibitor on the production by the liver of the CD salt. He based the concept on the observation that in patients whose bile showed a high level of D, there was very little of CD and, conversely, in those with much CD there was little D.

"And so," Heaton recalls, "there seemed to be an inverse relationship between the two, and Low-Beer was pursuing this as a purely academic exercise which, I must say, at the time I wasn't particularly interested in. And he was able to do some very sophisticated experiments using tagged bile salts which showed, beyond any doubt, that when you fed D to people you suppressed their liver synthesis of CD."

But it turned out that Low-Beer's academic exercise was not an academic exercise at all. And it turned out that way when news came from the Mayo Clinic in the States.

Remarkably enough, at Mayo investigators had discovered that the CD salt dissolves gallstones. They found that CD acts in the bile to increase its detergent properties relative to the amount of cholesterol present. With a high level of CD, the bile has spare detergent capacity and so, if a gallstone is present, the bile can leach the cholesterol out of the stone. (Currently, at many major medical centers in the U.S. and abroad, after very promising work at the Mayo Clinic with a limited number of patients whose gallstones were dissolved with CD treatment, intensive large-scale trials are under way, and if the efficacy and safety of CD treatment are proved out, many patients with gallstones may be spared surgery.)

"Now the Mayo work," Heaton points out, "would suggest that it is a good thing to have CD about in the bile. And if D displaces CD from the bile, as Tom Low-Beer's work shows it does, it might be a bad thing because you are removing a substance which in effect keeps the bile 'sweet.'

"And so, the question arose, if you feed D, does it actually make the bile into a bad detergent? Does the bile then, because D drives out CD, become more saturated with cholesterol?

"And, to our delight," Heaton says, "we found that that is indeed what happens." When cholesterol in the bile was measured in sixteen subjects before and after they were fed D, there was a significant rise in the cholesterol after the D feeding.

"Which shows," says Heaton, "that when you displace CD, you change the bile to create a gallstone-forming situation. And this is where we come back to bran."

With bran in the diet, there is less D to be absorbed from the colon and go back to the liver. The liver then increases the production of CD, and there is then more protective CD in the bile. The bile can handle its cholesterol content so that it is not so prone to crystallize out and form stones.

Moreover, it appears that with a high fiber diet the liver secretes bile that has less cholesterol content. In another study at Bristol reported in 1974, in six women with gallstones, feeding bran at an average rate of 47 grams a day reduced the cholesterol in the bile about 25 percent.

But how does all this jibe with an old axiom that gallstone formation is a disease of "fair, fat, and fortyish" women?

"That," says Ken Heaton, "is really an old wives' tale. It is true that obesity is associated with a high incidence of gallstones—and that is because overnutrition causes increased secretion of cholesterol into the bile. That is well documented by now.

"But gallstones have nothing to do with fair skin or fair hair. True, Scandinavians have a high incidence of gallstones, but the world's record is held by Pima Indians in Arizona.

"Women on the whole get gallstones at about twice the rate of men. They seem to have a propensity to put out a bit more cholesterol in their bile. This may well be a hormonal effect. It has not been adequately explained as yet.

"It doesn't mean that a woman is bound to get gallstones. An African woman on a native diet runs no risk at all. But being a woman in a gallstone-forming society makes you twice as liable as a man.

"Forty is rubbish. Gallstone formation is a disease which becomes increasingly common with age. And the most common age at which people present with gallstones is in the fifties and sixties. We did a survey in Bristol showing this conclusively."

Peter Cleave had thought that gallstones mainly arise from infections promoted by bacterial colonies in the colon. He had accepted the view of earlier physicians and surgeons that *E. coli* organisms from the colon were responsible, producing the infections in the biliary tract. The infection idea had been held by many and a distinguished physician, Lord Moynihan, had even enunciated an aphorism that every gallstone is a memorial to the bacteria entombed within it. Cleave had pinned the blame for the infections on an unnatural food surplus in the colon that fed *E. coli* bacteria so well that they multiplied out of hand. And the unnatural surplus was the result of a diet containing refined carbohydrates, which deceived the sensations of taste and satiety and led to overconsumption.

Peter Cleave is not a man who changes his mind easily. But Ken Heaton did change it. Heaton had marshaled what Cleave considered to be compelling evidence.

Overconsumption or overnutrition, in Heaton's view, is a potent cause of cholesterol secretion from the liver into the bile. It led to loading of the bile, supersaturating it, with cholesterol. And the overnutrition for the most part is traceable to refined carbohydrate.

And a refined diet also altered the physiology of the colon so that more D salt was formed and got back to the liver, which then produced less protective CD salt, with the result that the bile could not handle its cholesterol content well and was more likely to let it precipitate out and form stones.

Certainly, to the extent that bran lets less D get back to the liver, which then produces more CD, as studies with human volunteers have shown, and to the extent, too, that it reduces the cholesterol content of the bile, as studies with gallstone patients have demonstrated, it would appear to be helpful in minimizing the likelihood of gallstones.

Importantly, too, there could be a third way in which gallstones are induced by a refined diet.

Recently, several investigators have noted that in patients with gallstones, the total amount of the circulating bile salt pool is reduced. The cholesterol levels in the bile are high. And, beyond the reduced protective CD salt content, the whole bile salt content is reduced so that that, too, could encourage gallstone formation.

Notably, too, when artificial diets containing refined, fiber-depleted carbohydrates are used to induce gallstone formation in animals, the animals not only secrete bile that is loaded with cholesterol; their bile salt pool shrinks, too.

Recently, Heaton and his co-workers have been carrying out studies to see if bran, in addition to reducing the cholesterol content and increasing the protective CD content of the bile, might expand the total bile salt pool.

But bran has not done so.

That, to Heaton, is disappointing. But it is not altogether surprising. It hardly rules out the likelihood that eating an unrefined diet would be associated with an expanded and normal total bile salt pool.

"It would be naïve," Heaton says, "to suppose that adding bran to a refined diet really produces a situation fully equivalent to eating an unrefined diet."

12

"Turn it on its head, give it a bang..."

HOW much of a role might dietary fiber have in coronary heart disease and heart attacks and what could that role possibly be?

In 1956 Hugh Trowell had a most unusual patient. It was at Mulago Hospital at Makerere University in Uganda. The patient was an East African high court judge, forty-eight years old. His father had been a peasant in the Mbale district. The son became one of the first scholars at Nabumali High School, then worked as a teacher, a court interpreter, secretary-general of the African local government and, since 1951, had been a judge.

His diet had originally been native. But for the last twenty years it had been Western and plentiful. He had grown into a portly figure, quite unusual for an African of his tribe. When he was admitted to the hospital, he weighed 208 pounds and his height was only 5′2½″.

He had visited England in 1947, and while there had first noted some mild chest pain on walking and at times he had to stop and this quickly relieved his pain. Upon returning to Uganda, he had no more pain for eight years and then it returned. Again, it came on walking. Now it lasted five to ten minutes and was relieved by resting. He had a sense of constriction in his chest, but the pain did not radiate into the arm or neck. And then early in 1956 came a severe attack of pain while he was traveling in an automobile. It produced prostration. He was admitted to a local hospital and then transferred to Mulago Hospital the following day.

In all his years in Africa Hugh Trowell had not once seen such a case. But he had no trouble in diagnosing it and confirming the diagnosis with all the usual tests. The judge had coronary heart disease. Fortunately, he survived.

He became a historic patient—the first clinical case of coronary heart disease to be reported in East Africa.

Many things have been blamed for coronary heart disease—among them, excessive emotional stress, high blood pressure, and excessive cigarette smoking. And, of course, diet. It is widely agreed that coronary heart disease is probably not due to any single factor but rather may be the result of many factors—and that diet patterns matter a great deal.

One dietary factor that has had a tremendous amount of attention is saturated animal fat.

But could a fiber-depleted diet be an important factor that has been overlooked?

More than twenty years ago Alec Walker in South Africa—before he had met Denis Burkitt or Hugh Trowell—was one of the first to wonder about that.

At that time, as since, worldwide attention was focused on fats as the dietary factor involved in coronary heart disease. Fats raised cholesterol levels in the blood, and high levels had been found associated with CHD.

South Africa has a large Bantu population. Among the Bantu serum cholesterol levels are low. Not only do Bantus rarely suffer from such diseases as appendicitis and gallstones; rarely, too, are they victims of atherosclerosis and coronary heart disease.

Bantus in their villages eat relatively little fat. All told, their fat intake provides little more than a third of the proportion of calories that it does in Americans.

So—as Walker was reporting in the British *Lancet* in 1955—it is tempting to assign considerable significance to fat intake as the cause of high serum cholesterol and atherosclerosis and CHD.

But there were contradictory items of evidence, Walker noted, "which caution against attaching too much significance to level of fat intake per se."

For one thing, the fat intake of Eskimos is high, supplying over 40 percent of their calories. Yet, their serum cholesterol values are not abnormally elevated. Moreover, heart and blood vessel disease is almost unknown among these people and, for that matter, among the inhabitants of the Yukon who also have a high fat consumption.

For another thing, strict vegetarians have low serum cholesterol values despite their high fat intake. Three investigations, two in

Europe and one in the United States, showed that fat supplied 33, 34, and 35 percent respectively of vegetarians' calories.

Moreover, Walker's studies of the Bantu had impressed him with the fact that a low intake of fat was only one feature of their diet. Another was a high intake of dietary fiber. It seemed possible that diet with high fiber content might possibly bear some responsibility for low serum cholesterol values.

There were to be, as it were, other straws in the wind.

More than a dozen years ago a study in Belgium revealed that a group of Trappist monks aged fifty to sixty years whose diet contained 12 grams of fiber a day had a mean serum cholesterol of 195 (in milligrams per 100 milliliters, the standard way of measuring cholesterol blood levels). On the other hand, Benedictine monks of the same age, who ate 3 grams of fiber a day, had a mean serum cholesterol of 245.

In the United States there have been several studies of vegetarians. And in one, also done more than a dozen years ago, it turned out that a group of strict vegetarian men, mean age 51 years, who ate 23.9 grams of fiber a day had a mean serum cholesterol of 206, while another group of men, mean age 56 years, who ate the standard American diet, had a mean serum cholesterol of 288.

Leguminous seeds—beans and peas—are rich in fiber. In some parts of India, other countries in Asia, and in many countries in Africa the intake of chick peas and soya beans is high. And as long as fifteen years ago it was noted that where serum cholesterol levels were measured in these countries, they were low levels.

Whole rice has almost as much fiber (about 5 grams per 1,000 calories) as other whole cereal grains. If lightly milled, the rice has less fiber (about 1.4 grams per 1,000 calories). If highly milled and polished, the fiber content is greatly reduced (0.6 grams per 1,000 calories). It remains, however, an unbroken grain, and its starchy endosperm is intact. But when wheat is highly milled to make flour, most of the fiber is lost from the endosperm, too, being reduced from 0.7 grams to a mere trace. People who eat rice as a staple food get much more fiber than those who eat white bread and white flour. And in some countries in the Far East where poor inhabitants especially get as much as 70 and 80 percent of their calories from rice, there is far less coronary heart disease than among Western nations.

In the United States about twenty-five years ago, high blood pressure was treated with the Kempner diet of boiled rice, some

2,000 calories a day (with a fiber content of 1.4 to 10 grams), depending upon the degree of milling and polishing. Blood pressure fell, and the fall was ascribed to the very low intake of salt with the diet. But there was also a marked fall in serum cholesterol that was not explained. In a group of 284 patients treated for 90 days, the mean serum cholesterol fell from 257 to 192. Certainly, the reduced fat intake could have played a part but so might have the increased fiber intake.

In many parts of Africa, even today, coronary heart disease simply does not occur among blacks, and in other parts where it does, the incidence and severity is far from great.

In 1972 a study reported to the World Health Organization found that Nigerians' arteries "are smooth as velvet" and that coronary heart disease is virtually nonexistent, even in the bustling capital of Lagos. In a study in Ghana reported the same year it was noted that in Accra, with a population of 350,000, only ten patients with coronary heart disease were seen at the teaching hospital between 1968 and 1970.

In 1973 Dr. Walker could report that in Johannesburg there are less than 20 deaths per year among blacks, whereas in a local white population of the same age and sex structure, about 1,200 sudden deaths or heart attack episodes would be expected. It was not surprising. Earlier, two investigators looking for evidence of atherosclerosis among blacks in South Africa had done careful autopsy studies. They found that two-thirds of coronary arteries even in blacks past fifty at death showed no atherosclerosis at all and in the remainder the atherosclerosis was remarkably mild, consisting almost entirely of fatty streaks and small plaques, without ulceration.

Hugh Trowell pondered the rarity of the disease in Africans. In 1960 he was still very much fascinated by it when he wrote his book *Non-infective Disease in Africa,* in which he noted the rarity in Africans of other diseases, notably those of the bowel, which were common in westernized countries—diseases such as appendicitis, diverticular disease, ulcerative colitis, irritable colon, and polyps and cancer of the bowel. He considered then that Africans might be protected from the bowel diseases by their diet heavy in fiber. He wondered a bit whether such a diet might have some protective value against coronary heart disease and if so how.

When Trowell emerged from his retirement from medicine to work with Denis Burkitt, he was interested not only in obesity but also in coronary heart disease. Trowell was in his late sixties. He is today seventy-one, white-haired and with the look of a country vicar. He has a remarkable knowledge of medicine. Even as a vicar, he could not help but keep up with it and when, as a vicar, he regularly attended members of his parish who were in hospitals, he was often consulted by doctors in the hospitals on puzzling cases.

Hugh Trowell, with his tremendous intellectual curiosity and persistence, could, among other things, come up to London from his suburban home and check virtually the whole of medical literature on a disease, poring over it for hours at a time, and analyzing it, and sometimes, as he puts it, he would take a reported study, "turn it on its head, give it a bang, and see if the results which had been viewed one way might not just as well or perhaps better be viewed another way."

One of those studies was a classic one. It covered 1,154 age-matched Irish brothers, some of whom had remained in Ireland and some of whom had moved to the United States. The study was done in both Boston and Ireland. In Ireland only 29 percent of all deaths in men aged forty-five to sixty-four years are the result of coronary heart disease compared with 42 percent of all deaths in second-generation Americans in Massachusetts. This decreased incidence of the disease in Ireland was confirmed by a study of coronary arteries obtained from autopsies in Ireland. In these samples atherosclerosis occurred later and was less severe than in Boston.

Thorough physical examinations of the Irish brothers and the Boston brothers, including electrocardiographic studies, showed coronary heart disease present in about twice as many of the Boston brothers. The investigators expected that the Irish brothers would have lower serum cholesterol levels, and they did. But that was surprising when it turned out that the Irish brothers ate more total fat and more animal fat and less polyunsaturated fat. All this suggested that other factors must be operating in favor of the Irish brothers and their lower coronary heart disease rate and lower cholesterol levels.

But the intake of sugar, protein, and cholesterol, and also cigarette smoking and alcohol consumption, appeared very similar in the two groups, as were the blood pressures.

Curiously, too, the investigators noted that body weight was lower and skinfold measurements of body fat were lower in the Irish brothers. Yet, the Irish brothers ate food not only with a higher fat content but also a higher energy content, consuming

267 grams of starch per day compared with 116 grams for the Boston brothers. The Irish got the higher starch intake from cereal products and potatoes, consuming 30 percent more cereal products and 170 percent more potatoes than the Americans.

Perhaps increased physical activity in Ireland, especially in rural occupations, kept body weight normal despite increased intake of starch and fat. But if that were so, it did not explain the lower serum cholesterol levels. Very strenuous but not moderate physical activity offers some protection against coronary heart disease but does not reduce serum cholesterol levels.

When he analyzed that study, Hugh Trowell was quick to see what had been missed. Potatoes contain dietary fiber. The Irish brothers were getting 80 percent more dietary fiber every day than the Boston brothers. That had not been taken into account at all in the study. But it suggested to Trowell that the Irish brothers might well be getting protection against elevated cholesterol levels and obesity by their higher intake of fiber.

Trowell discovered there was reason to think so, considering a 1965 study that showed that when large amounts of potato were given in experimental diets, serum cholesterol levels were significantly reduced. The investigators then thought that fiber might be protective, but they had never gone on to develop the hypothesis.

Trowell was soon turning other studies on their heads and giving them rewarding bangs.

Many experiments have been performed on a variety of rodents fed different diets to determine the effect on cholesterol levels. But they have usually not considered the fiber content of the diets. Trowell did.

In one series of experiments rats were fed cholesterol along with one or the other of five different diets high in starch. Various preparations of rice starch, whole-ground rice, and tapioca starch were used for the diets. And the effects on cholesterol levels were strikingly different. They ranged from a high of 371 to a low of 130—very marked differences, indeed. There had not been any analysis or consideration of the fiber contents of the different diets. Trowell established that the diet that had produced the highest cholesterol level had the lowest fiber content, only 0.2 grams of fiber per 100 grams of food. On the other hand, the diet producing the lowest cholesterol level had contained the most fiber, 5.3 grams per 100 grams of food. And in between it was the same, the more the fiber content, the lower the cholesterol level.

Nobody had paid any attention to fiber. Nobody had known

anything about it. It simply was not considered important at all—an inert, unabsorbed ingredient, of no use and hardly worth paying any attention to.

Not only in animals but in humans as well, investigators had set out to determine whether leguminous seeds had any effect on cholesterol levels. Sure enough, they found that the seeds—one of the studies was in India and used bengal gram, a familiar bean there—lowered cholesterol levels. Leguminous seeds are about twice as rich in dietary fiber as cereal seeds, but none of the investigators considered that it might be the fiber that was bringing down the cholesterol. Some investigators had even considered the possibility that there might be some strange, unknown vitamin or other material in leguminous seeds, but they gave no thought to fiber.

What should have been an important study was published in a ridiculous place, an agricultural chemistry journal, and got virtually no attention. In South India Indian girls were fed high doses of cholesterol and their serum cholesterol went up. Then they were given high doses of cellulose. In a way, cellulose was not the right material to use because cellulose is not fiber but only a part of fiber. Yet, the serum choesterol of the girls fell.

The more he examined experimental studies of cholesterol levels in man and animals, the more Trowell found of reports in which, without having been recognized as such, fiber-rich starchy carbohydrates had reduced cholesterol levels in the blood and even cholesterol deposits in the coronary arteries.

One of the most bizarre instances of oversight came in a European study with forty middle-aged men. They had fairly high serum cholesterol levels, averaging about 250. Interested in determining which was responsible for pushing up the levels the most, white bread or sugar, the investigators first fed the men a lot of white bread, about 300 grams a day—and cholesterol levels went up. Next, they cut the white bread quantity back to 160 grams a day and used 140 grams of rolled oats, and cholesterol levels dropped, even to an average of about 223 after three weeks. Again, the white bread quantity was increased while the rolled oats were dropped, and cholesterol levels went up—and again when the bread quantity was cut and the oats added, the cholesterol levels came down. Immediately then, the bread and oats were cut back and now sugar was added to the diet. And cholesterol went up to about the same levels as with the bread.

"And there," says Hugh Trowell, "the experiment ended, with the experimenters evidently thinking, oh, dear, we planned these experiments to see if white flour pushes up cholesterol more than sugar, but they both seem to be equal pushers. Why didn't they look into the fact that rolled oats, which contain fiber, had brought the cholesterol levels down—down from about 250 to 233 in just three weeks, which is a big drop in three weeks!"

What could be the mechanism by which fiber reduces cholesterol levels?

One of the modern medications often used to bring down high cholesterol levels is a resin called cholestyramine. The material is not absorbed. It passes through the intestinal tract and is excreted in the stool—unchanged except for one thing. It has an affinity for bile salts. It latches onto them and carries them out in the stool.

And in both animal experiments and human trials dietary fiber has been found to do the same thing, increasing the excretion of bile salts.

Cholesterol goes into the manufacture of bile salts in the liver. And a possible explanation, which yet remains to be thoroughly documented, is that with increased excretion of the salts, the liver is called upon to produce more fresh salts, thus using up more cholesterol and leaving less of it to float around in the blood.

Fiber could have another value, too. Ongoing work by Dr. Kenneth Heaton at Bristol indicates that when fiber is present in the diet, there may be a reduction in the amount of cholesterol absorbed from the diet.

Denis Burkitt often makes a simple, terse statement, which sums up his philosophy of research. "If any cause has a number of different results, wherever the cause operates, the results will be found together. If you find the results together, suspect a common cause. It may not be, but suspect it."

It would be difficult to even think of two more dissimilar diseases than coronary heart disease and diverticular disease of the colon, and certainly they would hardly appear on the surface to be two results stemming from the same cause. Yet, Trowell was impressed by the fact that the two diseases were found together in more ways than one.

It was not only that both were common in developed countries and not in the developing.* It was also true that in northern Europe

* The rarity of both diseases in developing countries had been substantiated by reports obtained by Burkitt from 117 doctors in 135 hospitals in 20 African countries who stated that they had never seen a single case of diverticular disease and 94 had never diagnosed a single case of coronary heart disease. The Barag-

and North America where coronary heart disease is the commonest cause of death, diverticular disease is the commonest disease of the colon, found in 7.6 percent of English patients under the age of sixty years and in 34.9 percent of those over that age. And in Australia, where coronary heart disease is as frequent as in northern Europe, diverticular disease has been found in 40 percent of autopsies, while South African whites between twenty-five and forty-four years of age who have the highest prevalence of coronary heart disease in the world also show diverticula in one-third of their barium X-ray studies.

Moreover, it is not uncommon for the two diseases to occur in the same individual. In the United States a study of 840 autopsies reported in 1969 found a close association between the two. Another autopsy study in Australia reported the same year found severe atherosclerosis to have been more frequent in those who had had severe diverticular disease than in those in whom the colonic disorder had been mild.

Coronary heart disease is also closely associated with another disease—diabetes. The link between the two is now well documented.

One of the most revealing studies started in 1956 when Dr. Thomas Francis, Jr., and a University of Michigan research team persuaded 8,600 residents of Tecumseh, Michigan, nine-tenths of the community, to undergo complete physical examinations and blood and other tests. The objective was to study various factors influencing health.

Not only did the study find a high frequency of coronary heart disease among the known diabetics in the community; it also found that people with heart disease tended to have diabetes. It

---

wanath Hospital in Johannesburg, admitting some 40,000 Bantu patients a year, had recorded the diagnosis of coronary heart disease in only 30 Bantu patients in the last 11 years, most of them during 1971–1972; in the Pretoria Bantu Hospital, this diagnosis was recorded for a single patient in 1969, 3 patients in 1970, and 5 in 1971. Reports from 45 hospitals in the Indian subcontinent (India, Pakistan, Bangladesh, Nepal, and Burma) indicated that coronary heart disease had not been seen in 16 hospitals, and that only 18 hospitals had seen 5 or more cases of coronary heart disease a year. Most of the hospitals are in rural areas, and so it might be argued that the diseases might easily be missed where autopsies are few and electrocardiograms may not be available. Yet, the virtual absence of diverticular disease as a surgical emergency that often leads to death, and the infrequency of sudden death that could be caused by coronary heart disease even in a large series of autopsies in Uganda and at Groote Schuur Hopital, Capetown, confirms that the diseases are indeed rare in Africans.

even appeared that a high blood sugar level in an individual, whether a known diabetic or not, might be an important factor predicting the probability of coronary heart disease and heart attack.

At the Joslin Clinic in Boston 46.5 percent of deaths in diabetics has been found due to coronary heart disease. The famous Framingham study of 5,000 men and women (ongoing since 1949) in Framingham, Massachusetts, has found that among men aged thirty to fifty-nine initially free of coronary disease, diabetics subsequently developed 1.4 times the amount of heart disease as nondiabetics.

Hugh Trowell looked into diabetes.

Among other things, he found provocative data in what had happened to the death rate for diabetes in the female population in England and Wales over a period of years, before, then during, and after World War II. The rate had increased steadily from 120 per million women in 1931 to 153 in 1940. In 1941 it started to decrease steeply to reach the lowest level of the twentieth century, 86, in 1954. It remained fairly stationary between 1955 and 1959, but then began to increase steadily to 118 in 1970.

Trowell set out to identify the factor or factors accompanying and perhaps helping in the remarkable reduction in death rate.

We have already discussed the wartime changes made in flour milling. The ups and downs of discarding and retaining the part rich in fiber corresponded with the rise and fall of the diabetes death rate.

Other things, of course, had been happening. Fat consumption had undergone changes but they did not correlate with the changes in diabetes mortality.

Sugar was supposed to be a causative factor in diabetes. But sugar intake decreased by 25 percent in 1940 while the mortality rate was still increasing. Sugar intake was about the same as prewar in 1953 and went above those values in 1954, but the mortality rate continued to decrease.

One factor alone, the fiber content of flour, seemed to follow the same pattern as the mortality rate.

That did not constitute conclusive proof by any means that a high content of fiber in the diet was protective against diabetes. High extraction rates that leave more fiber in flour also increase the amounts in the flour of such nutrients as the vitamin biotin and the trace mineral magnesium.

Yet, it was notable that when there was a maximum increase in the fiber content of wheat flour, the largest reductions in diabetes mortality rates occurred.

Going back to World War I, Trowell found that in England in November 1916, a low extraction rate gradually increased to a high one in early 1918 but finished the year at the low of 1916. The diabetes mortality rate in women followed expectations exactly. Mortality rates for men changed along with those for women, showing less steep changes.

In the United States the high diabetes mortality rate—133 per million, both men and women—has largely remained stationary for many years. There has been no change in flour extraction and no experience with such a drastic fall in the mortality as that which occurred in Britain from 1941 to 1954 and from 1916 to 1918.

There were other suggestive studies. Various researchers in South Africa showed that among Cape Town Bantu who ate 6.5 grams of fiber per day, 3.6 percent had diabetes-like sugar level in blood tests, but among rural Transvaal Bantu who ate 24.8 grams of fiber a day, only five one-hundredths of a percent showed such sugar levels. Jews in Yemen customarily ate large amounts of whole-meal bread rich in fiber and had a low incidence of diabetes; with their immigration to modern Israel, however, the incidence shot up.

Trowell turned on their heads other animal studies, in which diabetes and obesity had been produced experimentally by varying diets without any attention being paid to fiber content.

These animals seldom developed diabetes or obesity when they fed, as they chose, on traditional foods: whole cereals for mice, fibrous vegetation for sand rats, fiber-rich leaves and shoots for monkeys. But when they were fed laboratory diets, many developed obesity and a condition resembling diabetes.

Trowell could readily figure out the amounts of fiber in both diets. Invariably, fiber was high in the traditional foodstuffs and very low in the laboratory diets.

However, Hugh Trowell is the first to agree that the mere association of any factor, such as fiber in flour, with declining human diabetes death rates such as had been observed in England during both wars does not prove a causal relationship. That can be demonstrated only by experiments in animals and man with starchy foods in which the dietary fiber content is known. The rechecking of previously done animal experiments provided some evidence. More such studies would be welcome. And in the present climate, with dietary fiber for the first time in history getting any real scientific attention, those studies undoubtedly will be done.

13

The sugar controversy

DENIS BURKITT and others who joined with him had started out tremendously stimulated and impressed with Peter Cleave's whole concept that assigned a major role to sugar as a provoker of diseases of Western civilization. As their studies proceeded, they had come to put somewhat less emphasis on possibly harmful attributes of sugar and much more emphasis on the beneficial effects of fiber.

Not that sugar, they felt, could or should be heavily discounted.

Cleave had not been alone in viewing sugar with alarm. Even as Cleave was attracting very little attention from either medical men or the lay public, Dr. John Yudkin of the University of London was attracting great attention and stirring up great controversy by viewing with skepticism the surging idea that increased fat consumption was clearly the culprit in the coronary heart disease epidemic; then he drew attention by announcing with considerable gusto that if you wanted to rely on the same kind of evidence used to incriminate fat, you could just as well incriminate the increased number of radio and TV sets, and by going on to make a case—which he maintained was far stronger and sounder—for indicting sugar.

John Yudkin is not only a physician; he is also a biochemist and a nutritionist—a not very common combination. He had started out with biochemical training at Cambridge. He was doing graduate work there in biochemistry, carrying out biochemical research and preparing to write his doctoral thesis on the research when, with the deepening recession in the early thirties, it occurred to him that it might be a good idea, as an anchor to windward, to study medicine. He went into medical training, completing his PhD thesis as he did so.

With a medical degree in hand, he had begun to do nutritional research at Cambridge, when the Second World War broke out. He went into the army, and there managed to do a little nutrition "when nobody was looking."

"Nobody," he recalls, "was interested in nutrition in relation to feeding the armed forces. In England nutrition was taken to be something any doctor could do more or less instinctively. We had nutritional experts in our war office, and they were just people in the medical corps who happened to be around when somebody was looking for someone to take charge of nutrition. So you had an awful lot of nonsense."

One such bit of nonsense Yudkin bumped into while serving in West Africa. He was in Sierra Leone in 1943, late in the war, when he encountered a common, persistent, puzzling, and unresponsive skin problem among African soldiers. It was not incapacitating, but it was highly irritating. The general belief was that it was an infection. It did not respond to any treatment.

It occurred to Yudkin that it might be a nutritional deficiency. It turned out to be an outbreak entirely due to a deficiency of the B vitamin, riboflavin. "It wasn't too difficult," says Yudkin, "to realize that some bright man sitting in the war office in Whitehall had devised what he called a 'West African Ration Scale.'" It was supposed to cover troops from all areas of what was then British North Africa stretching well over a thousand miles with intervals of French territory. All were supposed to eat the same food, although they came from tribes eating different foods.

Some were rice eaters; some customarily ate cassava; some millet. "As everybody ought to know," Yudkin says, "one thing people won't easily change is their staple. If you suddenly decreed that from tomorrow on all Americans should eat nothing but maize instead of bread, you can imagine what the reaction would be."

But the Sierra Leone troops who normally ate rice got rice in only one or two of the fourteen main meals of a week and were supposed to eat millet much of the rest of the time. To be sure, as Yudkin puts it, "you can sit down in Whitehall with pencil and paper and a book on the composition of foods, and you can figure out a diet adequate in all known nutrients, including riboflavin.

But if the riboflavin is mostly in the millet, and if you don't like and don't eat the millet, it isn't strange to relate that you don't get the riboflavin."

After the war, Yudkin was appointed to a chair in physiology at London University, where after several years he succeeded in setting up a department of nutrition that would become the major center for nutrition research in England.

Yudkin looked into the research that had been done correlating coronary disease with fat consumption. To him, it seemed to be based largely on incomplete epidemiological evidence.

In 1957 he published a paper intended to upset any seemingly glib assumptions that the case against fats had been proved. He announced that he had gotten together all the figures he could obtain from many more countries than ever before and that the fat hypothesis did not fit nearly as well as people had thought. It seemed to him that it might be possible to make at least as good an association between coronary deaths and sugar consumption.

He cautioned, too, that since coronary heart disease then was a disease associated with affluence, you could, if you were to rely solely on epidemiological information, pick virtually any characteristic of affluence and get an association, even including the number of television and radio sets in use in a country. Why not have a look at sugar and see if it fits as well as or better than fat, and go beyond epidemiology and have a look at experimental evidence, too?

"This thought," he says, "was greeted with deafening silence.

"And then about three years later, I began to think much more closely about man's eating behavior. What should diet be? In what ways has it changed? I wanted to know what were the changes that were induced by what I began to call the two dietary revolutions. The first was when man became a food producer—uniquely a food producer for there is no other animal that does something today in order to be able to eat next week or in a year's time. The second, an effect of the industrial revolution, was when man became technically knowledgeable and competent.

"It seemed to me that the nearer we got to what our preneolithic ancestors were eating, the more likely that we would be eating correctly. And if you are looking for a dietary cause of common diseases, of diseases that might be particularly associated with changes in diet, then you need to consider what are the major differences between current diets and the diets man used to eat.

"And reading around, reading Robert Ardrey, reading some of

the earlier paleontologists and anthropologists, and talking in South Africa with Raymond Dark, one of the early blokes who dug up man and did some early work that Leakey has been following, it seemed to me pretty evident that man used to eat a lot of meat to start with, whenever he could, and he ate shoots and young leaves, and probably dug up a root or two, and ate some fruit. He couldn't have eaten a very great deal of starchy foods because he can't digest raw starch, until he developed the controlled use of fire about a quarter of a million years ago.

"Then, about 8,000 to 10,000 years ago, he began to cultivate foods. And for fairly obvious reasons he began to be pushed into consuming these foods rather than animals to a greater and greater extent because animals are more difficult to produce, much more costly, and he had already left behind his hunting ability, and his population had grown because he had these greater amounts of foods from cultivation. So he got forced into the situation in which many poor countries today are in, depending upon a diet largely made up of cereal or root crops, largely starchy. Probably there wasn't much deficiency disease before that; there was death through starvation, but I'd guess there was no protein deficiency, no vitamin C deficiency, in the days when man was a hunter and food gatherer.

"The second dietary revolution, associated with industrialization, led to two new and different developments, both of them dependent on the fact that we now were so bloody clever with our science and developing technology.

"One was that we could rapidly increase food production because we knew how to drain land, irrigate it, cultivate it, use fertilizers, control disease—and then, later, we could use scientific genetics and new methods of food preservation. So total food availability, in spite of an increasing population, increased. The instinctive desire, if you like, for meat, which we had had to quell because meat had been so expensive to produce, could be met—first for wealthy people but gradually for the not so wealthy.

"Simultaneously, a completely different thing was happening. We began to be able to mess about with food. We were now able increasingly to make foods which the good lord never knew about. So that instead of being able only to produce more meat, more vegetables, more cereals, more fruit, we also were increasingly able to extract little bits from hither and thither and produce quite new things. And a large proportion of these new foods were rich in sugar—like ice cream, sweet drinks, confectionery.

"There were several reasons for this. We like sweet foods. Also, we were able increasingly to up our efficiency in extracting sugar from sugarcane and to breed cane with much higher yields. And a third reason lies in a whole range of very curious and unique properties of sugar. You can make boiled sweets, jams, with sugar; you can't make jams by boiling up fruit and adding saccharine. With saccharine, for example, you can make a sweet drink but then you're finished—and even the sweet drink tastes thin unless you put some sugar in. You can't make ice cream with saccharine; you can't caramelize, can't crystallize saccharine, as you can sugar. You can't dependably preserve fruits with saccharine as you can with sugar. You can't make chocolate without sugar.

"So the first big dietary change, 8,000 or so years ago, was a switch toward starch eating and away from protein eating. And the second, more recently with the industrial revolution, was the twofold one: an increase in God-given food plus a whole array of new foods, and the major component of the new foods was sugar.

"In the early sixties I wrote a paper on the role of palatability, what it has to do with what man eats. It considered that different animals eat completely different sorts of foods: a tiger is carnivorous; a cow is a grass eater; a giraffe eats acacia leaves and darn near little else and they have to be particular sorts of acacia leaves for he won't eat all sorts; a koala bear lives virtually on a dozen or so varieties of eucalyptus out of a hundred or so available varieties. Now the bear and the giraffe and the tiger and you and I get essentially the same nutrients out of a diet. We need them all with a few minor differences. The ruminant, for instance, can synthesize some things in his rumen that we can't, but by and large we all need the same things and yet eat different things. The cow licks her chops when she sees a luscious piece of grass that wouldn't make you or the tiger very excited.

"Palatability is in the picture, and it is more than the taste on your tongue; it's a matter of shape, color, and texture as well as flavor. And now man has the facility for making foodstuffs with all the desired palatability factors and without necessarily any relationship at all to their nutritional value.

"When somebody offers you a fruit drink, you expect that it should look like a fruit drink, have the color of one, the aroma, the sweetness. No manufacturer worth his mettle would refuse to make you a completely synthetic one that would meet your palatability demands. It may not have many vitamins or minerals or a number of other nutrients in it. But unless you're quite unusual, you're not concerned about nutrients; you're chiefly concerned about palatability, about the look and the taste of it, and of Coke drinks and the like, and you can bet that the sugar content is high.

"And by the early sixties I was saying that if there is a nutritional cause of diseases that is associated with affluence, then we certainly have to consider that a major characteristic of the diet of affluence is a very large amount of sugar.

"And then I went back and looked at changes in sugar consumption and discovered that in the early eighteenth century, 200 to 250 years ago, in this country, which was one of the early sugar consumers, we then consumed something like 4 to 5 pounds per capita per year; now we are consuming 110 to 120 pounds. Nothing else, nothing, has gone up in that sort of fashion.

"Now this doesn't necessarily prove that sugar is a cause of any disease that seems to be linked to diet, only that it may be worth looking further into. Except in perhaps the simplest diseases, epidemiology cannot prove the cause but only point to a possibility. You cannot prove that typhoid is caused by typhoid bacteria simply by going around and seeing that people sometimes get typhoid from drinking water. You have to isolate the bacteria and then find experimental ways to show it causes typhoid.

"So now we have to look for other evidence. But when it comes to coronary heart disease, you have a serious problem. Nobody is going to feed sugar to a group of people until they develop coronary disease. And the problem is complicated because none of the ordinary laboratory animals develop coronary disease.

"So you choose concomitants, associated phenomena, those things that people who get coronary disease also have. And, preferably, you don't choose just one, such as high serum cholesterol, for example, and say that anything that increases serum cholesterol is a cause of coronary disease and anything that lowers it is a preventive or cure. Rather, you consider that a number of phenomena are associated to a high degree with coronary heart disease—a high cholesterol level, yes; also, a high triglyceride level, high uric acid level, impaired glucose tolerance [as in diabetes], sticky platelets; also, frequently, hypertension and, often, obesity. And, working with animals, you see whether sugar produces any or many of this battery of phenomena.

"We have worked with several species of animals, and we have fed them different diets—one in which the carbohydrate is entirely or largely sugar, another in which the carbohydrate is entirely or largely starch. What I forgot to say before is that what has happened since sugar has come into our diet in these last couple of hundred years is that it has gradually replaced part of the starch; the total carbohydrate hasn't changed much but starch consumption has fallen and sugar consumption has risen and so the relevant experiment is one in which you compare these two carbohydrates.

"We have found differences in the effects of sugar between animal species. Sometimes you get something in one species and not in another, but mostly you get the same sort of things in varying degree. We have gotten increases in cholesterol and triglycerides—on the whole more easily in triglycerides. We have gotten impaired glucose tolerance. We have gotten sticky platelets, platelets that aggregate and clump more readily, and this is characteristic of atherosclerosis. We have gotten increases in uric acid. And in five species—rat, rabbit, pig, cockerel, and spiny mouse—we have produced straight, honest to goodness atheroma, fatty artery deposits.

"We have also done some experiments with human subjects, taking some starch out of their diets and replacing it with sugar, leaving everything else the same including total calories. They all have shown increases in fatty materials in the blood, in uric acid concentration, and in deterioration of glucose tolerance. And 30 percent also showed other things—a sudden increase in weight, about four or five pounds in two weeks, an increase in insulin in the blood, and platelet stickiness.

"We have used male students as subjects. And in our experiments we have pushed up the sugar enormously—from the national average of about 110 or 120 grams to 300 grams a day. If you think this is astounding, let me say there are people who consume 400 grams of sugar a day, and many who consume 300 or 350. Teenage boys here are the biggest consumers. Some of them eat a pound of sugar a day—in their frosted-sugar cereals to which they often add more sugar, their several cups of coffee with sugar in it, their Coke-and-bun midmorning breaks, and the other sugar-loaded foods and beverages they consume the rest of the day."

It seemed to Yudkin that another piece of evidence was needed. Could it be demonstrated that the man who eats more sugar stands a greater chance of getting coronary heart disease than the man who eats less sugar?

He questioned twenty men with coronary disease within the first three weeks after they had been admitted to the hospital with their first heart attack. Up to the attack they had had no hint that they had heart disease and had not consciously changed their diet. What had been their normal diet before they were taken ill?

Yudkin did the same thing with twenty-five patients with peripheral vascular disease (artery disease of the extremities) and with twenty-five matched control patients (with other than heart or artery ailments) for comparison.

He found a substantially higher sugar intake in the patients with coronary disease and with peripheral vascular disease than in the control subjects. The median values were 113 grams (about 28 grams to the ounce) of sugar a day for the coronary patients, 128 for those with vascular disease, but only 58 for the control patients.

Yudkin did a second study of the same type, this time using dietary questionnaires that patients could fill in. The median sugar intake in the coronary patients was 147 grams, about twice as high as for the control groups.

But other investigators could not duplicate Yudkin's dietary study results. In Toronto, Canada, a questionnaire survey of 170 military veterans, 86 with coronary heart disease and 84 age-matched controls from the same population of local veterans, found that the heart patients consumed slightly less sugar than the controls. In Montreal a study of 20 heart patients and 20 age-matched controls showed an average sugar intake for the heart patients of 121 grams a day and for the controls 117, an insignificant difference. In Dublin, Ireland, trained interviewers checked on 100 heart patients and 50 matched controls and found the average sugar intake of the controls was slightly higher, at 69 grams a day, than the average of the heart patients at 66.

Other studies also failed to show any great connection between sugar intake and coronary heart disease. The British Medical Research Council had a "Working Party on the Relationship between Dietary Sugar Intake and Arterial Disease" carry out studies in London and Scottish hospitals. In 1970 the Working Party reported that "the evidence in favour of a high sugar intake as a major factor in the development of myocardial infarction [heart attack] is extremely slender." The Party found that "the average sugar consumption was slightly greater in the patients with myocardial infarction than among the controls, but the differences were not statistically significant. Findings in one centre suggest that the slightly higher sugar intake in patients with myocardial infarction were likely to have been due to an association between the consumption of sugar and the smoking of cigarettes."

Peter Cleave and John Yudkin are not friends. But Cleave has offered a possible partial explanation of why Yudkin's sugar-coronary figures were not duplicated by findings of other investigators.

Cleave has always emphasized the importance of considering all forms of refined carbohydrate consumption: "Let us suppose that some investigator was engaged in a project, which at first sight would seem a sitting target, to relate obesity to the consumption of sugar. Surprisingly, someone opposing such a relationship would have no trouble at all in turning the tables on the investigator, for he would be able to assemble a collection of the fattest men in any town, who did not have a sweet tooth between them, and in consequence consumed very little sugar at all. These people would represent the formidable army of beer drinkers in this country—people who, in their tastes, prefer the bitter to the sweet. And the reason the beer often causes extreme obesity lies not in its content of alcohol (which substance, of itself, when taken to excess, causes wasting), but in its content of malt sugar. Indeed, through the presence of this malt sugar (which is not a sweet sugar), beer becomes a perfect example of a refined carbohydrate. This case shows the importance of relating any manifestation of the saccharine disease to the consumpton of *all* forms of refined carbohydrates and not only to one form. For all of them end up substantially as glucose in the blood. This crucial point partly explains why Yudkin's findings of a high sugar consumption in coronary sufferers has not been confirmed by other investigators and in particular by a Medical Research Council Working Party."

Cleave differed from Yudkin. Yudkin put all his emphasis on sugar. To Yudkin, heavy consumption of sugar was a major, direct cause not only of coronary heart disease but also of diabetes. It led to diabetes because, as Yudkin saw it, sugar stimulated the pancreas to release insulin—at first. But then with continued high sugar intake, the pancreas begins to wear out.

Yudkin also saw excessive sugar intake as being related to severe indigestion or dyspepsia in many people because of an irritating effect on the lining of the upper gastrointestinal tract—the esophagus, stomach, and duodenum.

For Cleave the problem lay not just with excessive intake of sugar itself but also with excessive intake of other refined carbohydrates, most particularly white flour, which, while taken in as starch, rapidly became converted to sugar on digestion.

Cleave saw obesity and diabetes and coronary heart disease all as the result of overeating, with the overeating caused by the unnatural concentration present in white flour and sugar, which deceived the appetite so that it no longer properly regulated food intake.

Cleave considered fiber to have some importance. It was fiber's removal by refining that made for the concentration. And it was the removal of fiber that also led to constipation and such complications of constipation, as he saw it, as varicose veins and hemorrhoids.

And appendicitis, gallbladder disease, and diverticular disease Cleave saw arising from the hordes of microbes subsisting on the unnatural food surpluses in the gut resulting from overeating.

Denis Burkitt and those who worked with him started out with Cleave's emphasis on sugar and his somewhat lesser emphasis on dietary fiber. But as they proceeded, they reversed that emphasis. They saw the outstanding characteristic of the modern Western diet to be the decreased consumption of all fiber-rich starchy foods —cereals, potatoes, and leguminous seeds—and the replacement of these with smaller amounts of fiber-depleted starchy cereals—white flour and polished rice. And they conceived of starchy foods undepleted of fiber as being protective against many diseases.

But sugar was not to be disregarded. All of them viewed with much misgiving the present high level of sugar consumption in Western nations.

And recent U.S. research adds still another reason for concern over excessive intake of sugar along with other refined carbohydrates. The research points to the importance of a metal, chromium, found in small amounts in unrefined carbohydrates but largely lost from the refined.

Chromium appears to be required along with insulin for the proper handling of sugar in the blood. And just as a deficiency of insulin can produce diabetes with its excessive blood sugar levels, so, animal experiments now indicate, does a deficiency of chromium.

Moreover, Dr. Henry A. Schroeder of Dartmouth Medical School has shown in repeated animal studies that chromium deficiency encourages the laying down of fatty deposits in arteries (atherosclerosis).

Schroeder's studies also indicate that adult Americans generally have only half as much chromium in their bodies as adult Africans. Yet, most of us are born with a good chromium reserve, which becomes depleted with age.

Why the depletion? Quite normally, when we eat carbohydrates

—both sugar and starches, the latter being split in the intestine into sugars and absorbed as such—the sugar level in the blood rises. In response the pancreas sends an increased supply of insulin into the blood and, at the same time, chromium is mobilized from body stores and moves into the blood to work with the insulin in handling the sugar.

Quite normally, too, when the job is done, the chromium in the blood circulates to the kidneys where about 20 percent of it is excreted in the urine.

As long as the sugar and starch in the diet contain chromium, enough of the metal can be absorbed into the body to make up for the losses in the urine and there is no net loss.

But if the sugar or starch or both contain very little chromium, there is a net loss from the body, and chromium stores are depleted more and more over a period of time.

The fact is that the sugar and starch most commonly used in Western diets are very low in chromium.

Raw sugar has a rich supply of the metal, some 36 micrograms per 150 grams. But refined white sugar contains only 3 to 4 micrograms per 150 grams. Schroeder has calculated that that amount of refined sugar taken daily could cause a net loss of about 8.75 milligrams of chromium in the urine in a year, more than the total body content, so that essential chromium would have to come from other foods.

But white flour is also chromium deficient. While whole wheat contains 175 micrograms of chromium per 100 grams, refined white flour contains only 23. So white flour, Schroeder reported, may cause depletion of body chromium just as does refined sugar.

It, therefore, appears to Schroeder that the typical Western diet, with so many calories coming from refined sugar and refined flour, could hardly have been better designed to provide as little chromium as possible and to deplete body stores of it by not replacing urinary losses.

If anyone wanted to deliberately develop atherosclerosis, according to Schroeder's studies, one could do no better than what many people do—drink many cups of coffee throughout the day, all loaded with three or four teaspoonfuls of sugar; use toasted white bread laden with marmalade or jam along with processed breakfast foods laden with sugar; eat sandwiches on white bread and a slab of pie for lunch; and more white bread, or polished rice, and maybe a slab of lemon meringue pie for dinner followed by a sticky sweet liqueur or two. "Such a diet will almost surely result in an elevated serum cholesterol, a depletion of chromium, and atherosclerosis."

Not long ago, in a book entitled *The Trace Elements and Man,* Dr. Schroeder remarked that the most effective way to lick the atherosclerotic-diabetic syndrome is by prevention. "To this end," he wrote, "I look to the day, although I may never see it, when this essential micronutrient (chromium) so necessary to the integrity of the arteries is either not removed from our major sources of calories by refining, or if the public insists on white flour and white sugar, is restored in sufficient quantities to those foods to ensure their adequate metabolism.

"Modern man," Schroeder added, "makes many mistakes through lack of knowledge, but there is no excuse for his continuing his mistakes in the face of knowledge."

14

The fiber story is much more than a bran story

MANY people may be tempted to take an oversimplified view of dietary fiber and to think that all they have to do to put our refined, low fiber diet right is to add bran to the diet.

But that, indeed, would be naïve.

True, the arrival of a small amount of bran, the outer fiber-rich part of cereal kernels, once or twice a day in the colon might benefit certain disorders of the colon, such as constipation and diverticular disease.

But bran, even in large amounts if it could be tolerated, would not provide the other benefits that a fiber-rich diet appears able to afford.

For one thing, bran would not necessarily alter the amount of food consumed, and the problem of overnutrition would remain virtually untouched.

For another, bran would not affect the rate at which carbohydrates are absorbed as would a fiber-rich diet, and the rate is of no small consequence.

Carbohydrate—starch—is formed always within the walls of plant cells. The digestive system of man secretes enzymes that digest starch, but the cell walls are resistant to these enzymes, and it is the skeleton of these walls that is dietary fiber.

A major constituent of the walls is the most abundant organic compound on earth—cellulose—which literally supports most of the living things on earth, which happen to be plants. Cellulose is the unique component—missing in animal cells—that allows plants to grow stiffly upright, away from the earth, and toward the sun. All plants, from ferns to redwoods, have this common unit of support.

There are numerous other constituents of the cell walls, and thus of dietary fiber, among them materials called lignins, others called pentosans, still others called pectins, and others besides.

When plant material is processed by the miller or sugar refiner and the "nutrients" are extracted from it, what is left in the pipeline is fibrous material. It is called bran and beet pulp respectively, and it has been and continues to be fed to animals.

Adding bran to the diet does, indeed, put back some of the fiber that has been refined out of it. But it does not put it back as it was, surrounding the carbohydrates.

When you consume carbohydrate with the natural fiber still surrounding it, it is quite a different matter from when you consume white flour and add on bran. As Hugh Trowell likes to put it, "It is no good having the package a few hours later if you want to stop the eggs from being cracked."

With the package intact on unrefined carbohydrate foods, as Ken Heaton observed, they require chewing; they demand to be chewed. Because of the chewing requirement, it takes longer to eat unrefined carbohydrates, and that is one natural obstacle to overconsumption. With the fiber package intact, you are also eating a food, part of which is nonnutritive, is not absorbed, and does not supply calories. The fiber has a space-filling effect, and that is another obstacle to excessive intake. And with the space-filling effect of both the fiber and the increased saliva and gastric juice flow stimulated by the chewing, you feel full on less calories. There is a natural satiety effect.

Nor do the important effects of the natural fiber package stop there.

With fiber surrounding the carbohydrate, the digestive enzymes cannot diffuse through so readily to digest the starch. And the increased bulk provided by the fiber speeds up transit time so that there is less time for the processes of digestion and absorption. And it is notable that the effect is not only on the digestion and absorption of carbohydrates, but also on the digestion and absorption of energy from protein and fat. Many studies have shown that while out of a typical modern, refined diet 93.2 percent of the available energy in the foods is absorbed, the absorption is cut to 88 to 89 percent when whole-meal bread and other unrefined carbohydrate foods are substituted for the refined. And Dr. David

A. T. Southgate of the Dunn Nutritional Laboratory at Cambridge, one of the world's top authorities on fiber, has shown in studies with young men and young women that as the amount of unrefined carbohydrates in the diet is increased, the digestibility of protein drops from 92 percent to as low as 85 percent and of fat from 97 percent to as low as 93 percent.

The rate of absorption of carbohydrates is significant in more ways than one. When carbohydrate is turned into sugar and absorbed rapidly, the pancreas responds with a big surge of insulin to take care of the relatively sudden high load of sugar in the blood.

One effect of such a surge is to change metabolism in such a way that synthesis of fat from the sugar is promoted. Another effect at the same time is to promote the entrance of that fat into cells. "Which means," says Heaton, "that if you have a surge of insulin after a meal, you are more likely to lay down fat than if you don't have the surge. You can take the same amount of carbohydrates, either as refined or unrefined. But while the fiber-depleted refined carbohydrates will be absorbed rapidly and may cause a big surge of insulin secretion and the laying down of fats, the same amount of unrefined, fiber-rich carbohydrates will be absorbed slowly, occasioning only a slow, steady release of insulin, with little fat laid down.

Moreover, Heaton adds, a big surge of insulin also affects the liver, causing it to secrete into the blood more cholesterol and triglycerides.

This last fact may be a reason why animal studies have demonstrated that bran added to the diet is far less effective than an equal amount of fiber in whole cereals in reducing serum cholesterol levels.

15

Fiber as protection against toxic effects of food additives and drugs

DOES fiber provide protection against toxic effects of food additives and drugs, and may the lack of it help to make these compounds hazards to health?

That possibility has been raised recently by Dr. Benjamin H. Ershoff, a research professor of biochemistry at Loma Linda University and the University of Southern California. He has mustered evidence from extensive animal studies—his own and those of others—that it may be a serious possibility.

No extensive discussion is needed here about the increasing concern over the possible contamination of the internal environment of the human body by the widespread use of food additives that have no nutritional value but might have potential for doing harm. On the average, each of us consumes in the course of a year about three pounds of chemicals that are not normal constituents of foods. Some of these—preservatives, coloring agents, and sweeteners—are deliberately added to food; others, such as insecticides and antibiotics, may get there unintentionally.

As for drugs, during the past thirty years many new, powerful, and effective agents have been developed and have largely replaced traditional types of "natural" remedies such as medicinal herbs and preparations made from them. With most traditional remedies, the dangers of side effects were slight. But side effects of modern effective drugs are hardly a small problem.

For example, Dr. Kenneth L. Melmon at the University of California Medical Center at San Francisco in 1973 found that

3 to 5 percent of all admissions to hospitals under study were due to illness caused by drugs, and that 30 percent of the patients had further adverse reactions from drugs given to them during their hospital stay; also, these drugs almost doubled the duration of their hospitalization.

Ershoff points to many studies conducted during the past twenty years that indicate the beneficial effects of plant fiber-containing materials in counteracting the toxic effects of a number of drugs, chemicals, and food additives when administered to animals fed on low fiber diets.

Actually, the first clue came as far back as 1943 when two American medical investigators observed that immature mice who were being given a compound related to Vitamin C—glucoascorbic acid—developed a severe condition characterized by growth failure, diarrhea, hemorrhages beneath the skin, hair loss, and death. But the condition developed only in mice who were being fed on a highly refined ration. It did not develop at all in mice fed similar doses of glucoascorbic acid in conjunction with a natural food stock ration or in mice fed the refined diet supplemented with dried grass.

In 1954 Ershoff showed that alfalfa meal when incorporated in the diet was similarly effective in counteracting the toxic effects of glucoascorbic acid. Painstakingly, he continued to see if any known nutrient in the alfalfa meal might account for the phenomenon. It was not a nutrient that was responsible. When juice was extracted from the alfalfa, it had no effect. But the pulp remaining after the juice extraction worked.

It turned out that various grasses—rye, orchard, wheat, fescue, and oat—were also potent sources of the active factor. When cellulose alone was tried, it had a moderate protective effect, considerably less than that obtained with the fiber-containing alfalfa and varied grasses.

In 1953 other investigators reported that a compound called Tween 60 when given to rats fed on a low fiber diet induced growth retardation, diarrhea, and other toxic effects, but these could be counteracted if at the same time bulk-forming substances such as celluflour or agar were added to the diet. Subsequently, Ershoff tried various bulk-forming substances, found marked differences in their effectiveness, tried cellulose and found it less than satisfactorily effective. But alfalfa meal worked—and it worked on a whole series of other toxic compounds.

Then Ershoff experimented with a human drug, a diuretic called chlorazanil hydrochloride. The medication has been used effectively in the United States and Europe in patients with edema or waterlogging resulting from congestive heart failure, toxemia of pregnancy, peripheral vascular disease, cirrhosis of the liver, kidney disease, and other conditions. In some patients, however, it produced an undesirable effect, an increase in nitrogen levels in the blood.

Ershoff fed immature rats a high toxic level of the drug in a low fiber diet and got an increase in blood nitrogen. But with the addition of alfalfa meal and other plant fiber-containing materials, the blood nitrogen rise was counteracted.

In 1972 Ershoff went on to cyclamate, a sweetener. When cyclamate was incorporated at a 5 percent level in a low fiber diet and fed to immature rats, the animals showed a marked retardation of growth, an unthrifty appearance of the fur, and extensive diarrhea. When alfalfa meal was also incorporated in the diet, the animals' fur appeared smooth and sleek and with the exception of a mild diarrhea the rats seemed normal. Other plant fiber-containing materials such as wheat bran and desiccated kelp also had a protective effect. And Ershoff went on to find that still other such materials did as well, including Irish moss powder, watercress powder, parsley powder, celery leaf and stalk powder, carrot root powder, and pectin, which is a material from apple pulp and the rind of citrus fruits.

In 1974 Ershoff became concerned about the human health implications.

All the studies indicated that various drugs, chemicals, and food additives that could be highly toxic when fed to rats and mice in conjunction with low fiber diets had no deleterious effect when fed with diets high in dietary fiber.

He was now very much aware, too, of the reports by Denis Burkitt, Hugh Trowell, and others that, as the result of the refining of flour and other cereals and the increased consumption of sugar at the expense of bread, there had been a marked reduction in fiber in the diet of Western man. In addition, there had been a marked decline in the consumption of fresh fruits and vegetables, which are also sources of fiber, and an increased consumption of fruit juices, which are virtually devoid of fiber. The dietary fiber intake of Western man was now estimated at about 20 percent of what it was in the mid-nineteenth century and what it is for the rural African today on his native diet. And associated with the dietary fiber reduction in the West, there has been an accompanying increase in diverticular disease, polyps and cancer of the colon, hemorrhoids, and still other disorders still virtually nonexistent in people living on high fiber diets.

Are there even more disorders associated with the fiber reduction?

It seemed to Ershoff that there might well be, that "in view of the low fiber diets ingested by so many persons in the United States and other Western countries, serious questions arise as to whether the ingestion of drugs, chemicals, and food additives that may be without deleterious effects when ingested by persons on high fiber diets may not constitute a hazard to health for a substantial portion of the population of these countries."

16

Now where do we stand?

MANY changes have occurred as man has become sophisticated. Certainly diet alterations have been many. Protein consumption has risen. Total carbohydrate intake has fallen. While carbohydrate supplied by sugar has increased manyfold, less bread and other cereal foods are eaten and what are eaten are almost wholly of refined white flour. Fat intake has increased. While fat supplies 10 percent of calories for rural Africans, the proportion is 35 to 45 percent in the United States, England, and other Western countries.

All these changes have come under study—all except, until very recently, one: the change in fiber content of the diet.

Fiber is undigested. It has no nutritional value. It seemed logical to pay it no attention as having any possible role in maintaining health. In fact, it was viewed largely as a contaminant, and its removal has even been believed to enhance the quality of food.

But if it is a contaminant—a totally unfortunate term—it is clearly an essential contaminant.

"Can I give you an illustration?" says Hugh Trowell.

"The air is our environment. We breathe in air. And it has in it available air, which we call oxygen, 20 percent. And it has unavailable air, which is called nitrogen, 80 percent. And we and our ancestors have breathed this environment in those proportions for 400 million years, since life came out of the ocean.

"Now I am told by people who are experts that you could cut the nitrogen in air from 80 to 40 percent and increase the oxygen from 20 to 60 percent, and you could breathe such air as normal air and get away with it. But if you start cutting the nitrogen below half its normal figure, 40 percent, you run into trouble. In a premature baby you produce a serious eye disease. You mightily increase the hazard for ordinary people who, not adapted to such a proportion of the gases, develop new bacterial colonies, and many of them will be dead of pneumonia within a few weeks. An anesthetist who can juggle the mixture of oxygen and nitrogen is always careful not to give pure oxygen to anyone for very long.

"Now, similarly, we believe that we have eaten cell wall, which is dietary fiber, for 500 million years, since life started in the ocean. And we have always eaten it in a certain proportion because we were basically vegetarians, plant food gatherers.

"Only about a century or two ago did we say, 'Boys, let's really get the "goodness" out of the cell contents; we can forget about the cell walls.'

"And we believe that this is a very big change in terms of evolutionary adaptation. And that people who eat plant cell wall as my African patients did because they got the food out of the garden every day and other people who eat this in other parts of the world have a very different incidence, a tremendously lower incidence, of diseases than we 'goodness' eaters who have tossed away plant cell wall; and they have that lower incidence exactly because they haven't yet been exposed to our 'goodness,' our very civilized and highly refined 'goodies.'"

That, in a nutshell, is the fiber hypothesis. How well does it hold up?

An old tale—true—has it that Charles Darwin observed that only bumblebees with their long tongues could pollinate red clover effectively and that the prime enemies of bumblebees are field mice that devour both larvae and honeycombs. The better crops of clover near villages, Darwin remarked, had much to do with the control of mice by the village cats.

But another scientist went further, suggesting that since red clover was the staple diet of British cattle and bully beef the staple of the British sailor, a relationship might be shown between British naval victories and keeping cats.

Diseases, too, have relationships—much closer ones— and it has often been rewarding to ferret out these relationships.

Malaria and mosquitoes, cholera and contaminated water, lung cancer and tobacco smoke—these are examples of associations that have clarified causes and even made possible preventive measures.

Establishing relationships between symptoms also can be rewarding. Skin rashes, penile lesions, palate perforation, bone changes, and aortic aneurysms or balloonings out—observations that some or all of these conditions tended to occur together in the same patients led to the realization that they were manifestations of a single disease, syphilis, and a common cause.

The fiber hypothesis, of course, takes into account relationships—relationships, one with the other, of many common, troublesome, some of them deadly, diseases that at first blush, would seem to be entirely unrelated; relationships of time and place, of increased prevalence; and relationships with concomitant environmental changes.

All are relatively new diseases. Coronary heart disease was considered a rarity by Sir William Osler in 1910 and was still newsworthy in 1925 when an English physician, Sir John McNee, described with some excitement two cases of this "rare condition" he had seen in the United States. Appendicitis was first described in 1812 and appeared to become common after 1880. Diverticular disease has become a major problem only in the last fifty years; hiatus hernia only in the last thirty years; hemorrhoids and tumors of the colon also appear to be recent developments; so, too, gallbladder disease, which has increased by 350 percent since 1940 in the records of the Bristol Royal Infirmary in England.

All these diseases, while common in all economically developed countries, are rare or unknown in rural Africa and all less-developed communities.

Moreover, not only are they geographically related; they are chronologically related. Where the incidence of one begins to rise, so does that of the others. Where, for example, diabetes surges upward, so later does appendicitis. Atherosclerosis and lesions of the colon then become common after another generation or so. With migration, too—from Africa to America, from Japan to America, and from country to city in Africa and Japan—these diseases become much more common.

And, beyond sharing geographical and chronological relationships, these diseases often occur in the same individuals. Most notable is the strong tendency for atherosclerosis, obesity, and diabetes to occur in individual patients.

The most compelling argument for relating these diseases to a fiber-depleted diet, of course, was the great rise in their prevalence after the removal, in the latter part of the last century, of most of the cereal fiber still remaining in Western diets.

Admittedly, this was only one dietary change. But rational explanations of how lack of fiber may cause the various diseases could be presented and, as we have seen, have been.

Is it an open and shut case, proved beyond all doubt, that lack of dietary fiber is the sole cause, or the major cause, of all these diseases?

Hardly.

Not one of the men who are studying fiber and its relationship to disease would say that.

"Nearly all disease," says Denis Burkitt, "has more than one causative factor. Not in any of these diseases would I suggest that fiber deficiency is a sole causative factor, merely that it may be one important factor. What I would emphasize is that a fiber-depleted diet is a common factor, common to a number of characteristic Western diseases. It is a major factor, I believe, in some, a less important factor in others, but it is common to each of them and offers the only reasonable explanation put forward, I think, why these diseases are associated.

"I like to do everything with little pictures," Burkitt says. "I want to draw a picture—a little flask for each of these diseases. When the flask overflows, we can say, disease begins. The overflow would come from pipes leading into the flask.

"It may be that for some diseases—for example, coronary heart disease and diabetes—there are many, many pipes and for others, fewer. And the pipes may vary in size. But one pipe would be fiber-depleted diet. That pipe may be a very big one for diverticular disease. It may be very big for appendicitis. It may be a smaller pipe for coronary heart disease and diabetes. But that pipe would be there, common to all these characteristically Western diseases."

Because he has what he calls his "platform"—his renown in the medical profession for his lymphoma work—Burkitt is listened to when he talks at medical meetings. And all the more so because he emphasizes, as does Hugh Trowell and all the others who have been associated with him, that what he is presenting is a hypothesis about a dietary factor long overlooked but now certainly worthy of thorough investigation. He welcomes to the investigation any evidence in favor or against the hypothesis.

There are skeptics. In fact, to some, the very simplicity of the concept is offensive, as if only complicated explanations are likely to have any validity and simple ones none. Of them, Burkitt is likely to ask calmly, "But what alternative hypothesis do you have to explain the epidemiology and interrelationships of these diseases?" There isn't any as of now.

Burkitt has aroused interest. So have Trowell, Heaton, Painter, and others with their journal papers and talks. And in the last three years or so there has been a mushrooming of research on fiber and its role in health—and on fiber itself: what it actually is and how many kinds of it there are. That research is going on now in many centers in England, the United States, and elsewhere in the world.

And that is exactly what Burkitt and his "fiber gang" want and are happy to have.

Many specific research projects could be valuable. They are not easy to do, and even as recently as a year or two ago would have had little chance of getting done. But with the rapidly growing interest, they could well be undertaken soon.

Alec Walker has suggested several projects. One would be to select from questionnaire surveys people who clearly are habituated to a higher-than-average intake of whole-grain products and lower-than-average intake of refined carbohydrate foods. Then it would be possible to determine what the prevalence was among them of the various diseases believed to be associated with low fiber diets. If it were found to be much lower than for the population as a whole, that would count heavily in favor of the fiber hypothesis.

Another, suggests Walker, would be an experiment done with a random group of about 500 men, between 30 and 39 years old, who would be willing to include 15 grams of bran (about 2 heaping teaspoonfuls) in their daily diet for an indefinite period. Measurements, such as for bowel motility, constipation incidence, overweight, blood sugar and cholesterol and triglyceride levels, would have to be done at the start of the study, after six months, and after a year. In addition, studies on bile salt excretion and on bacterial colonies in the stools would be needed. Subsequently, investigations would be needed to learn if the beneficial effects achieved with bran could be further improved by reduction in the intake of refined carbohydrate foods, including sugar.

With these and other studies it would become possible to determine the minimum changes in diet needed to demonstrably lower the prevalence, or delay the onset, of the various diseases.

Fiber itself certainly needs study. It has long been surrounded by mystery, ignorance, and confusion.

It is a very complex substance. It consists of celluloses, of which there are thousands of different physical varieties. It also contains hemicelluloses, which got that name because they were once thought to be precursors of cellulose but now are known to have standing in their own right and are known also to consist of varied substances. And there are, as well, pectic substances and lignins. Some peptic substances are in apple pulp and the rind of oranges, for example, and are often used by food processors for gelling purposes. Lignins are "woody" like materials.

No food table in the world even now contains a full analysis of all the fiber present in food. Food tables record only crude fiber. But crude fiber is not what we encounter. It is only the portion of total fiber that resists and is not dissolved out of food by acids and alkalis in laboratory determinations. But acids and alkalis dissolve out hemicelluloses which, in wheat, for example, are three to four times the weight of crude fiber.

There is confusion indeed. Recently Hugh Trowell suggested that a new term be adopted—and it largely has been—dietary fiber. It includes all the fiber, crude plus the rest. And roughly speaking, in many cereals dietary fiber is five times the figure for crude fiber.

It is all this dietary fiber not just the crude—the whole group of cell wall remnants—that remains intact in the small intestine and passes to the large bowel.

Only recently have there been any attempts to analyze what differences exist in the various dietary fiber components in various foods. Such analysis is far from simple and until more work is done, only a few broad generalizations can be made. Thus, plant cell walls eaten before maturity, such as occur in leafy cabbage and soft immature green peas, have little lignin, but much cellulose. Mature solid fruits, such as the apple, and fleshy tubers, such as the potato, have approximately equal proportions of hemicellulose, cellulose, and lignin. Cereals contain a large amount of hemicellulose and, when mature, also contain a fair amount of lignin.

Already, it has become evident that the components of dietary fiber have different properties. Cellulose, for example, acts as a moderate water adsorbent in the bowel. Some of the other components such as hemicellulose are strong adsorbers. And water adsorption counts in making the stool moister and softer. Lignin, however, does not adsorb water to any significant extent, but there is some evidence that it does latch onto and bind bile salts to carry them out in the stool.

Undoubtedly, there are other differences in properties between the components of dietary fiber—and they could be significant differences. Many experimental studies have been done with bran to determine the influence of dietary fiber. But bran is a mixture of all the above components, and it is impossible to tell from the use of a mixture which particular component is responsible for any particular valuable effect. What are needed are intensive studies carried out with isolated components.

"As more work is done," says Denis Burkitt, "I think we may well find that the dietary fiber situation in the beginning—now—is much like the situation with B vitamins. At first, there were values attributed to the complex of B vitamins. Then came the studies that assigned specific values to the individual B vitamins—B_1, B_3, B_6, B_{12}, and the others. Similarly, I think, we may find specific values for the individual components of dietary fiber."

And that might mean that different plants, and even the same plants at different ages, could be analyzed for their specific arrays of fiber components, and diets might be based on overall optimal assortments of cereals, vegetables, and fruits, and perhaps even optimal assortments for individuals with specific problems or tendencies.

Actually, some of this work is being undertaken by David Southgate and his group at the Dunn Nutritional Laboratory at Cambridge, and it is almost certain that more will be—and more, in fact, may already be—undertaken at other institutions.

17

Practicalities for the reader

IT is not, as you see, open and shut. There is going to be much more to come on dietary fiber.

If the hypothesis is further substantiated, it would be no exaggeration to predict that the effect on the health of Western nations of a return to a high fiber diet would be much more beneficial than the elimination of cigarette smoking.

That return, in some ways, might be easier for many than the elimination of smoking.

In determining whether it is a return you wish to consider, you will, of course, use your own judgment in evaluating the existing evidence.

It seems to many informed physicians and scientists now that certainly more evidence is desirable but what is available justifies a return.

In the United States five scientists, four of them physicians, are calling for action by doctors, nutritionists, public health officials, and the federal government to increase the use of fiber in the American diet.

In a "white paper" on fiber and health, the five men—Dr. William O. Dobbins, director of the division of gastroenterology at George Washington University Medical Center in the District of Columbia, Dr. Franz Goldstein, chief of gastroenterology at Lankenau Hospital in Philadelphia, Dr. Daniel H. Connor, chief of the geographic pathology division of the Armed Forces Institute of Pathology, Dr. Stuart Danovitch, a Washington, D.C., gastroenterologist, and Michael Jacobson, Ph.D. co-director of the Center for Science in the Public Interest in Washington—review the evidence.

They conclude that increased consumption of dietary fiber would be a "prudent preventative measure," that "enough is known to justify informing people that a diet richer in unrefined plant products and thus higher in dietary fiber would increase the health of almost everyone."

They urge that the U.S. Department of Agriculture, which reaches millions through its extension service, school lunch, school breakfast, and food stamp programs, encourage consumption of fiber-rich foods through its TV spots, publications, press releases, and authority to approve foods used in its programs; that the Department of Defense, which buys and serves vast quantities of food, inform servicemen, civilian employees, and their families of the health benefits of whole-grain products, bran, legumes, fruits, and vegetables; that the Department of Health, Education and Welfare encourage food editors, consumer writers, authors of cookbooks, schoolteachers, and medical school professors to inform their audiences of the value of fiber and whole-grain foods.

In England in 1974 the Technology Assessment Consumerism Centre—based at Manchester University and set up "to help find a way through the maze of technological systems in which we have lost ourselves"—issued an eighty-four-page report on "Bread: An Assessment of the British Bread Industry," in which it took "the lid off the bread bin."

Noting the evidence on the importance of fiber, it also noted that fiber has been eliminated from white bread "with increasing skill and completeness." That where whole-meal flour has 100 percent of the fiber, a 90 percent extraction flour has 50 percent of the original fiber content, and the now-standard 72 percent extraction flour used to make the white loaf has less than 8 percent of the original fiber.

"The industry," said the report, "has concentrated its economic and technological effort into the production of a nutritionally inferior loaf. More and more people are phasing bread out of their diet, indicating that the baking industry has failed both the consumer and itself. Instead of mounting expensive promotional campaigns for products of dubious social value, such as 'slimming' breads or part-baked loaves, they would be advised to disseminate more accurate and understandable nutritional information, and to encourage the consumption of whole-meal bread."

Not surprisingly, in the homes of Denis Burkitt and many others researching fiber, fiber has been restored to the diet.

How is that achievable?

Basic Guidelines

About carbohydrates—refined and unrefined. The most important energy source in the human diet, carbohydrate occurs in two forms. One, of course, is starch—composed of large complex molecules—which is, in fact, a plant's energy store. The other is sugar—made up of small relatively simple molecules. Among the well-known types of sugars are sucrose or cane sugar, fructose or fruit sugar, and glucose or dextrose, the latter being the form in which all sugar is absorbed into the blood. Starch—tasteless, incapable of dissolving in water—seems far removed from sugar; yet, in fact, it is converted to sugar in the intestinal tract before being absorbed into the body.

Unrefined carbohydrates are carbohydrates in their natural form; they may be cooked but they are not otherwise processed. In the natural state carbohydrates are never isolated and "pure." Instead, they are mingled with other materials. Without exception, starch is associated with protein, various vitamins and minerals, and with indigestible fiber, as in cereals such as wheat and rice and various vegetables. Sugars, too, in nature are always associated with fiber. Moreover, except in the case of honey, sugars in nature are in dilute form so that, for example, a fairly large sweet apple will contain only a teaspoonful of sugar.

Natural, unrefined carbohydrates provide vitamins and other nutrients, take chewing, tend to be filling, and are the only sources of dietary fiber.

On the other hand, refined carbohydrates—white flour, white rice, and sugar—are the products of the milling of flour that involves the use of steel rollers to pull out the starch-rich portion of the grain and of the extraction of sugar from sugar beet and cane.

For adequate restoration of fiber to the diet, it is necessary, as much as possible, to eat natural, unrefined carbohydrates and avoid the refined as much as possible.

Although it is possible to keep on consuming the usual large quantities of refined carbohydrates and restore some or even much or all of the refined-out fiber by using bran as a supplement, that, as we have seen earlier, is not the same thing as materially increasing the unrefined carbohydrate intake. One very important reason is that as the intake of unrefined carbohydrate is increased, the apparent digestibility of other constituents in the diet is decreased—a good thing in our overconsuming society.

About cereal fiber and vegetable fiber. Both are important. It appears from recent research that cereals contain fiber that is more resistant to digestion than that of many vegetables and fruits, and therefore more remains to function effectively throughout the gastrointestinal tract. Thus, there are grounds for considering cereal fiber as something special. But, again, other fiber as well is needed.

About wheat germ. The wheat grain is a tiny seed, which if left alone, will grow into a new plant. The grain has three main parts. The bran—somewhat like an eggshell—protects the softer inside. Unlike an eggshell, however, it has important roles in diet, providing dietary fiber and also vitamins and minerals. The endosperm of the grain, similar to the white of an egg, is largely protein and starch. Finally, there is wheat germ, the germ of the seed which, like the yolk of an egg, is rich not in fiber but in nutrients, including vitamins and minerals.

For use as a flour, wheat grain is crushed. Different kinds of flours can be produced, depending upon the extent to which various parts of the grain are removed or retained. These flours are differentiated by their extraction rates, indicating amounts of grain retained. Whole-meal flour, with 100 percent extraction rate, contains all the ground grain. White flour, now commonly of 70–72 percent extraction, retains only the endosperm, with both germ and bran removed.

With both germ and bran removed, there is a huge loss not only of fiber but of vitamins and minerals. According to a 1971 study * by Dr. H. Schroeder of Dartmouth Medical College, the losses are as follows:

NUTRIENT	LOSS IN FLOUR (IN %)
Thiamine (Vitamin B_1)	77.1
Riboflavin (Vitamin B_2)	80.0
Niacin	80.8
Vitamin B_6	71.8
Pantothenic acid	50.0
Alpha-tocopherol (Vitamin E)	86.3
Calcium	60.0

* *American Journal of Clinical Nutrition,* May 1971, Vol. 24, pp. 467–69.

Phosphorus	70.9
Magnesium	84.7
Potassium	77.0
Sodium	78.3
Chromium	40.0
Manganese	85.8
Iron	75.6
Cobalt	88.5
Copper	67.9
Zinc	77.7
Selenium	15.9
Molybdenum	48.0

No attempt is made to restore most of these nutrients to white flour. So-called "enriched" white flour has returned to it usually only vitamins B_1, B_2, niacin, and iron. While the use of bran as a supplement provides some unrestored nutrients, those from wheat germ would still be missing. And the use of wheat germ supplement along with bran supplement still would not provide the values of eating carbohydrates whole and unrefined.

Understanding the confusion of food tables. If you happen to look at tables of food composition, you will find indications of fiber content. But they are not true indications.

The figures are for crude fiber—what is left after a carbohydrate is treated with acid and then with alkali, which dissolves some of the previously unrecognized important constituents of fiber.

We have seen that dietary fiber—which is what counts—consists of crude fiber *plus* these other vital constituents, known technically as celluloses, lignins, pentosans (hemicellulose), and pectic substances. Dietary fiber is what survives, not when a carbohydrate is boiled up with acid and alkali but after it is mixed with human digestive juices, and it is this fiber, not crude fiber, that does its work in the digestive tract.

Thus, in a table of food composition as in the Appendix, you will find the crude fiber content of whole wheat recorded as approximately 2 grams per 100 grams. But whole wheat dietary fiber content ranges from 15.3 to 18.1 grams per 100 grams, seven to nine times as much as mere crude fiber.

And you need to take that into account—and adjust accordingly—when you consider listings of crude fiber for various foods.

A start now is being made toward developing food composition tables that will accurately reflect true dietary fiber values—and, in fact, values for the various constituents of dietary fiber. But the required analyses are difficult, time-consuming, and expensive, and still lie in the future.

Must a high fiber diet be boring and restricted? Not at all. Virtually all real gourmet foods and delicacies can be used.

Knowing what to eat and what not to eat. The objective is to eat, as much as possible, natural, unrefined carbohydrates in place of the refined, that is, white flour and all things made with it, and refined sugar.

Any change of diet in that direction is helpful. The greater the change, the better. But the change can be made gradually, and you are likely to be motivated to make greater and greater change as you begin to experience what lesser changes provide.

How much fiber? Exact requirements are not definitively established. Yet, there are useful guidelines.

Rural Africans—healthy, nonobese, very largely free of such problems as constipation, diverticular disease, cancer of the colon, diabetes, coronary heart disease, and other chronic afflictions of westernized peoples—take in about 25 grams of crude fiber daily (28 grams are roughly equivalent to 1 ounce). They get about 13.5 grams of it in cereals, 6 grams in potatoes and legumes, 5.3 in fruit and vegetables.

On the other hand, studies in the United States and Britain indicate an intake of only about 6.4 grams of crude fiber daily. In the United States that is made up of 0.5 grams of cereals, 0.9 grams of potatoes and legumes, 5.0 grams of fruit and vegetables. In Britain, it is made up of 0.5 grams of cereals, 1.4 of potatoes and legumes, and 4.5 of fruit and vegetables.

Almost all Africans south of the Sahara eat natural carbohydrates or lightly processed cereals. In South Africa corn (maize) is the principal cereal eaten by the Bantu, and the most popular variety (Impala special) contains 1.4 grams of crude fiber per 100 grams. Millet, the traditional cereal of Africa, is still consumed by many and contains 4.5 grams of crude fiber per 100 grams.

In tropical Africa starchy staples predominate. Although they contain more moisture than cereals, they do provide a fair amount of fiber: for example, sweet potatoes, 9.0 grams of crude fiber per 1,000 calories; tapioca, 7.0 grams; plantains, 2.5 grams. And leguminous seeds and groundnuts, which are common foods, are rich sources of fiber.

Before 1890 in both Britain and the United States, it is estimated that each individual consumed daily about 450 grams—15 ounces, almost a full pound—of bread and got from it about 1.5 grams of crude fiber. But today's bread, made of highly refined flour, contains only a small fraction of that fiber content, and the amount of bread consumed has fallen to less than one-third the amount consumed in 1890, so that fiber intake from this source has probably declined on the average by more than 80 percent. There has been a reduction, too, in consumption of cereals in porridge and other forms high in fiber, so that all told cereal fiber intake today is only one-tenth of what it was in 1890.

How much fiber, then, should be restored to the diet?

Excellent results in relieving common colon disorders—including constipation, spastic colon, and diverticular disease—have been achieved with the use of 10 to 15 grams (½ ounce; 15 grams are roughly 1 heaping tablespoon) of bran and 200 grams (6⅔ ounces) of appropriate fruit and vegetables such as carrots, apples, oranges, and brussels sprouts. (More later about suitable fruit and vegetables.) The 15 grams of bran contain the same amount of fiber to be found in about 75 grams (about ⅔ cup) of whole-grain wheatmeal—and, for reasons we have noted before and will again later, greater reliance on the wheatmeal (and there are many ways to use it) than on bran is to be preferred.

That amount of fiber restoration, suggests Dr. Martin Eastwood of the University of Edinburgh, might well be universally adopted.

You are very likely to know when you are getting a suitable amount of fiber by the effects on the stools: they will become softer, well formed, and readily passed without straining.

Does that mean more calories? No. By replacing as much as possible refined carbohydrates with unrefined, you are not going to be adding calories to your diet. If anything, by such substitution, you are likely—even as you get the fiber you need—to be taking in less calories for reasons presented in Chapter 10.

Foods to find substitutes for: white bread, rolls and cakes, biscuits, and puddings made with white flour, sugar, molasses, honey, or syrup; white polished rice; ordinary spaghetti, macaroni, and other pastas; most commercial breakfast cereals. Also, as much as possible, sugars (white, brown, molasses, honey, syrup), and candies, sweetened desserts, sweetened beverages, sweetened fruits, condensed milk, and sweetened yogurts.

Foods to eat freely. Many foods, of course, contain no carbohydrates, and there are no restrictions on them in terms of a high fiber diet. They include cheese of all kinds; meat of all kinds, including poultry and game and liver and sweetbreads; fish of all kinds, including shellfish; fats and oils such as butter, margarine, and vegetable oils; clear soups and homemade soups thickened with such vegetables as potatoes and lentils; all spices, herbs, and condiments; preserves such as unsweetened chutneys and unsweetened pickles.

And carbohydrates to eat freely. There are many (see below).

Specific Positives

With much in the way of noncarbohydrate foods to choose from, there is also much in the way of natural, unrefined carbohydrates, some of which you may find immediately enjoyable even if you have not tried them before, and others for which you may develop a taste.

You can start the day, as much as possible, with freshly squeezed orange juice. Cut the oranges in halves, pick out the pits with tip of knife, then squeeze. Do not sieve it but retain all the pulp.

Add a bowl of fiber-rich cereal. You can choose from a number available: oatmeal, the old-fashioned, slow-cooking kind, not the "instant" ("instant" anything can generally be counted upon to be more highly refined than its less convenient counterpart); or a whole-grain wheat cereal preparation designed to be cooked; shredded wheat; cereals labeled as being all bran or made up of a goodly percentage of bran. And, rather than adding sugar, add apple, banana, or other fruit.

Flour

Where you now use white flour and products made with it, use instead as much as possible true whole-meal flour—whole wheat or whole rye that is 100 percent extraction. (Much so-called whole meal is not made of whole-grain flour, so do look for 100 percent extraction labeling or inquire about the extraction—from the manufacturer if necessary.)

Bread

Instead of white bread, use bread made from whole wheat or whole rye flour (100 percent extraction). Note that many brown breads are by no means whole meal. So do not go by color alone but establish—by means of labeling or inquiry—that the bread is, in fact, made from whole wheat or whole rye flour.

Whole-meal bread helps keep you slim; it contains 7 percent fewer calories than white bread and most brown breads.

You can, if you like, make your own whole-meal bread and even an extra high fiber bread, a bran-plus loaf, which is enjoying increasing popularity in England.

Many good cookbooks—among them, the classic *Joy of Cooking*—contain varied recipes for making whole-grain breads.*

For the bran-plus loaf (whole-meal bread with extra bran), the ingredients are: 8 cups unsifted whole-meal flour, 100 percent; 1 cup unprocessed bran (obtainable at moderate cost in health food stores and possibly in some supermarkets); 3½ cups lukewarm water; 1 teaspoon brown sugar or honey; † 1 tablespoon (or ¼-ounce package) dried yeast; 2 teaspoons salt.

Mix salt with flour and bran. Mix yeast with sugar and add ½ cup water. Leave for 10 minutes to froth up, then pour into flour and add rest of water. Mix well and knead for 5 minutes. Put into bread tins and leave to rise for about 1½ hours. Bake in hot oven for 40 minutes.

Pastry and other high fiber recipes

From the dietetic department of the United Bristol Hospitals in England come two well-tested recipes and suggestions for other high fiber dishes, in addition to the bran-plus loaf.

Pastry. The ingredients: 2 cups unsifted flour, 100 percent whole wheat; ½ cup fat; pinch of salt. Rub fat and salt in flour. Add water to mix and knead lightly to a fairly wet dough. Roll out and bake as required in 450-degree oven for 20 minutes, then lower to 375 degrees until cooked. For fruit pies, brush surface with milk and sprinkle on a little brown sugar. (See the bran-plus loaf footnote regarding the use of sugar.)

Apple crumble. The ingredients: 1 pound apples; ¼ cup or a little more sultanas (white raisins); 1 cup unsifted whole-meal flour; 6 tablespoons butter or margarine; ¾ cup loosely packed

---

* "We have become so accustomed to our highly bleached white flours," *The Joy of Cooking* points out, "that we forget that earlier cooks knew only whole-kernel flours. You may substitute 1 cup of very finely milled whole-grain flour sometimes called whole-kernel or graham flour, for 1 cup of all-purpose flour. For coarsely ground whole-grain flour, substitute 1 cup for 7/8 cup of all-purpose flour. This is stirred lightly rather than sifted before measuring. Yeast breads from whole wheat flours do not have to be kneaded. They can be mixed and allowed to rise just once in the pan. If kneading is omitted, the texture will be coarse."

† As you become accustomed to less sweetening of all foods (see "The matter of sweets," p. 136), you should find it possible to modify recipes calling for sugar, molasses, or honey by using less and less amounts. You may even from the beginning substitute raisins and other fruits containing natural sugars.

desiccated coconut; ¼ cup brown sugar (see bran-plus loaf). Prepare the apples and slice and place in a greased fireproof dish in layers with the sultanas. Rub the butter into the flour. Add the coconut and sugar and continue to rub until the mixture forms very small lumps. Spread evenly over the apples and bake for approximately 30 minutes at 400 degrees.

Other cakes, biscuits, and scones. As an alternative to whole-meal bread, if you enjoy baking, try making cakes, biscuits, and scones using whole-meal flour, fat, and eggs—and adding, for variety and interest, spices, dried fruits and nuts; for example, dates, figs, currants, raisins, sultanas, ground almonds, walnuts, Brazil nuts, coconut, cinnamon, nutmeg, ginger, mixed spice.

Using whole wheat flour in place of cake flour or all-purpose flour, you can make rolled biscuits and biscuit sticks.

There are many other possibilities. For cakes and biscuits with high fiber content, you do not have to depend entirely on whole wheat flour. You can use oatmeal or rolled oats with dried fruits and nuts.

If you like muffins, you can make them by using 1⅓ cups whole-grain flour along with ⅔ cup sifted all-purpose flour, 2 tablespoons molasses (see bran-plus loaf), 1 teaspoon salt, 2 teaspoons double-acting baking powder, 1 egg, 1 cup milk, 2 to 3 teaspoons melted butter (adding ¼ cup chopped dates or raisins if you like), and mixing and baking as usual for muffins. Or you can omit the all-purpose flour and use instead 1½ cups whole-grain flour.

You can also make bran muffins, using 2 cups whole-grain flour and 1½ cups bran, along with 2 tablespoons sugar and ½ cup molasses (see bran-plus loaf), ¼ teaspoon salt, 1¼ teaspoons baking soda, 2 cups buttermilk, 1 beaten egg, 2 to 4 tablespoons melted butter. You can add if you like 1 to 2 tablespoons grated orange rind, or ½ cup mashed bananas, or 1 cup nutmeats and raisins.

If waffles, griddle cakes, and French toast happen to be favorites, you can make them, too, with whole-grain products. For griddle cakes, prepare as usual but use half the customary amount of cake flour and substitute whole-grain flour for the other half.

Similarly, you can use whole-grain products for producing pizzas, tortillas, and the shells for enchiladas and tacos.

Popovers. These too can be whole grain. Use much the same recipe as you usually do—1 cup milk, 1 tablespoon melted butter, ¼ teaspoon salt, 2 eggs—but then, in place of the usual 1 cup all-purpose flour, use just one-third that amount and add ⅔ cup whole-grain flour.

Meat dishes. You can use whole-grain bread or whole-grain bread crumbs in place of white bread or white bread crumbs in many dishes—for example, in preparing ground beef for meat loaf, hamburgers, hamburger casseroles, and German meatballs; in chicken, veal and lamb patties; and in such other dishes as stuffed cabbage, sauerkraut balls, and pork balls in tomato sauce.

Breading. For breading meats and fish you can use whole-meal flour instead of refined, and whole-meal bread crumbs (or, if you prefer, bran) instead of white bread crumbs.

Thickening. For thickening sauces, stews, etc. you can use whole-meal flour again instead of refined flour or cornstarch, and, again, whole-meal bread crumbs (or, if you prefer, bran) instead of white bread crumbs.

Rice. Use brown (unpolished) rice if you can. Brown rice, which retains its bran coat and its full complement of vitamins (not all are restored by any means to polished rice), is slower to tenderize than highly polished rice and may take about twice as long to cook but is very much worth it.

Whole-meal spaghetti and macaroni. Use these in place of the routine kind. If they—and brown rice as well—are not available elsewhere, they may be found in health food stores.

(As the demand for high fiber foods and ingredients begins to rise, they will undoubtedly become increasingly available in all types of food stores, including supermarkets.)

Peanut and other nut butter. Peanut butter is, of course, very popular. Yet, smooth and delicious as commercially prepared peanut butters may be, they are often not made of intact nuts. Nuts contain fiber. Their valuable germ portions, as in grains, contain minerals, vitamins, and proteins. Yet, both fiber and germ content may be diminished in some commercial peanut butters as a means of keeping them from becoming rancid as the result of the heat of processing and storage.

You can make your own full-bodied peanut butter in an electric blender, using fresh roasted or salted peanuts and adding 1½ to 3 cups bland oil such as safflower or vegetable oil for each cup peanuts.

You might want to try blending other nuts—such as walnuts, cashews, and almonds—into nut butter, retaining their germ and fiber values.

Seeds and berries. Seeds such as whole sesame seeds and sunflower seeds (see the chart following the Appendix), along with such seed-filled berries as raspberries, blackberries, and loganberries provide dietary fiber. So do seaweeds (which can be purchased ready to eat in packages found in Oriental retail food stores).

Fruits and vegetables. As much as possible, eat all kinds in generous amounts, preferably raw or cooked only lightly. Potatoes should be boiled or baked in their skins. If possible, eat them with skins intact. They are no more fattening than any other natural food. Uncooked dried fruits also may be used, especially figs (see chart).

It is important to remember that cooking, particularly when you prepare fruits and vegetables, tends to break down fiber—and the more cooking, the more the breakdown.

Certain fruits and vegetables appear to be particularly valuable. At the University of Edinburgh, Dr. Martin Eastwood has made a special study of varying values of fruits and vegetables.

Eastwood began with the thought that a lot of things had been happening to fruits and vegetables. That many "modern" types had been developed for succulence, for canning potential, for freezing potential—and nobody had ever cared about the fiber content since fiber was not even mentioned in the nutrition books.

"And, of course," he remarks, "fiber content and succulence do not go together. The sort of vegetables one's grandfather grew in his allotment of garden would be different from the ones we have which are grown for succulence and canning and the like. And I suspect, though this is unproven, that Victorian fruits and vegetables may have been more fibrous than contemporary ones because geneticists and agriculturists have bred for everything but fiber."

Eastwood and his colleagues looked at twenty-six fruits and vegetables for their physical characteristics. "We looked at factors which could affect bowel function. We looked to see how they swelled in water because the more they swelled, the more water they picked up, as bran does, the more they might benefit bowel function. And we got a pecking order of swellability."

Eastwood found that, next to bran, mango was highly swellable, but mango is not a commonly eaten food in the West.*

The ranking order of the twenty-six fruits and vegetables in terms of their water-holding and swellability characteristics is as

* You might want to try mango. A delicious flattish oval fruit, when chilled and eaten raw, it can be rich and sweet but never cloying.

follows, with bran at the head of the list and turnip last in order: bran, mango, carrot, apple, brussels sprouts, oatmeal, aubergine (eggplant), spring cabbage, maize, orange, pear, green bean, lettuce, winter cabbage, pea, onion, celery, cucumber, broad beans, tomato, cauliflower, banana, rhubarb, old potato, new potato, turnip.

"We could now," says Eastwood, "start talking to patients about how to increase fiber in their diet with selected fruits and vegetables, giving priority to the first group."

Another word about fruits—as much as possible the skins should be eaten for their fiber content.

A special word about the lignin in fruits and vegetables. Lignin, as we have seen earlier, is one of the constituents of dietary fiber. It is a peculiar one—the only one, at least the only one so far determined, that is not actually a carbohydrate. (Technically, it is what is known as an extremely complex aromatic polymer.)

Lignin is under increasingly intensive study—and for good reason. And that is because of the evidence—far from definitive as yet—that a diet rich in lignin may increase bile salt excretion in the stool, which, as we have seen, is valuable.

Yet, the lignin content of the diet in the United States and Great Britain, Dr. David Southgate found, is very low, often at a level where it is very difficult to measure at all precisely.

The fact is that lignin tends to form as plants mature. Many foods eaten by man have not been analyzed for their lignin content. But it is known that soft, immature cell wall structures contain only small amounts—for example, plantains and bananas, 2 percent; immature peas, 7 percent; cabbage, 6 percent. Fully matured cells and cereals contain more: apple, 25 percent; potato, 32 percent; and wheat, 23 percent.

Generally, the more woody the tissue, the more lignin. "But we tend to discard most of the woody tissues," says Southgate. "They are mostly pared away; we don't eat very heavily lignified tissues at all. In most vegetables one would tend to take off the outer leaves, which are the older leaves, and the lignin content goes up with age. One tends to cut out the hard stalks of cabbages and things like that. And one doesn't eat very mature carrots; when carrots mature, they get quite lignified."

Given the present limited knowledge of the effects of lignin, no one is prepared to say that there should be heavy concentration on increasing the lignin content of the diet. But it might not be amiss to pay a little attention to it, to get some of it in such foods as apples and potatoes and wheat, and perhaps to be a little less generous in discarding outer leaves and possibly even stalks wholesale.

The matter of sweets. Drs. Cleave, Yudkin, and Heaton put considerable emphasis on avoiding sugar as much as possible and all the sweet things containing it. Burkitt and others might be said to be somewhat less concerned but nevertheless are in favor of a reduced intake.

As Dr. Cleave sees it, the ideal solution to the problem of eating excessive amounts of ordinary sugar lies in substituting natural sugar, by eating raw fruit or dried fruit. "For example," he says, "instead of sweetening a rice pudding with sugar, eat a banana or two with it, or make the pudding with some raisins. The substitution of raw fruit involves little or no loss in pleasure, but it does involve some extra expense."

You may find it difficult to believe, Yudkin says, "but when you really have gotten used to taking very little sugar in your foods and drinks, you will notice that all your foods have a wide range of interesting flavors that you had forgotten. Swamping everything with sugar tends to hide these flavors, and blunts the sensitivity of your palate. You will especially notice how much you enjoy fruit, all the subtle differences between one sort of apple or pear or orange and another. And unless you eat a couple of pounds or more of fresh fruit a day, you can't possibly get to eat as much as the average person now eats of refined sugar, let alone the amount that so many people eat. All this does *not* mean that you must never, in any circumstances, take a piece of pie or a helping of ice cream. No great harm will come to you if, at a dinner party, you accept something special that your hostess has made for the occasion. Eating sensibly is not the same as making a nuisance of yourself."

Dr. Heaton has a set of suggestions he gives to patients on how to learn to live happily with a markedly reduced sugar intake: try and lose your taste for sweetened foods, and though you can expect that this will take time, after a while you will find that foods containing only natural sugar—all fruits and even milk and carrots—taste surprisingly sweet.

Aim to give up sugar completely in coffee and tea. If you are accustomed to taking several teaspoons in a drink, you may need to cut down gradually. For example, from 2 to 1½ teaspoonfuls immediately; after two weeks, to 1 teaspoonful; after another two weeks, to half a spoonful; then, to a quarter; and then, to none at all. And it is not advisable to use artificial sweeteners because they prevent you from losing your taste for sweet things.

At times when you are accustomed to eating sweets or chocolates, eat instead fresh fruits such as apples, grapes, bananas; dried fruit such as raisins or figs; nuts; raw carrots or celery.

If you drink alcohol, Heaton suggests, remember that spirits contain no sugar, but tonic water, ginger ale, bitter lemon, etc. do. Choose dry wines and sherries rather than sweet. Bitters contain maltose, a sugar, but small quantities may be permissible.

And honey, he advises, although a natural food, is a refined sugar —refined by bees for bees. If you miss eating much honey, jam, and other preserves, try a small amount of homemade coarse marmalade that uses little sugar.

If you need to reduce weight. As noted in an earlier chapter, for many reasons the restoration of dietary fiber can help significantly to control overall food intake. Indeed, with white flour and sugar avoided and fiber restored, says Dr. Cleave, "the appetite can again be allowed to regulate the amount to be eaten, as it is designed to do, and we can ignore any question of calories, just as all creatures in the wild state ignore them (and they never suffer from overweight)."

For the removal of excess weight already present, a certain amount of going a bit hungry may be necessary. But it is almost certainly likely to be much less work and much more permanently successful with the restoration of dietary fiber.

What of bran? The pros and cons of bran, as indicated earlier, need special consideration. Bran is not a panacea, though there is a temptation to regard it as such.

Unprocessed bran has its uses. But except in special cases, it may not be needed.

Bran can be used for constipation. It can be used effectively for diverticular disease. But even for these problems, it is not essential. "It is probable that both these conditions are deficiency diseases due to lack of natural fiber," says Dr. Neil Painter. The best way of correcting this deficiency is to eat plenty of fresh fruit and vegetables, and to eat whole-meal bread and to use whole-meal flour.

"Often the poor," he notes, "cannot afford enough fresh fruit and vegetables. They can correct for this lack of roughage by adding unprocessed bran to their diet. Bran tastes like sawdust and is difficult to take dry. It should be washed down with water, fruit juice, or milk. It may be sprinkled on cereals, mixed with soup, or with flour in baking." *

More about bran—a recent study by Dr. Eastwood and his associates at Edinburgh indicates that not all brans are equally efficacious. Coarse bran appeared to be much more effective than fine bran, they found, in reducing pressures within the large bowel and in reducing transit time. Bran with coarse particles held more water than did fine bran.

"The whole problem is not bran, it is dietary fiber," Eastwood wrote me as this book was being prepared. "The evidence does not support any idea that bran is the sole panacea. The diet of Africans, against which comparisons are made, never has contained bran, and I think that it would be misleading to further this view."

Denis Burkitt, too, wrote: "I am increasingly convinced that Dr. Trowell is right in emphasizing the need for a diet from which the fiber has not been removed rather than merely adding lost fiber requirements."

If protection is to be gained from dietary fiber, not alone against constipation and diverticular disease but obesity, diabetes, and coronary heart disease, it will come not so much—in some conditions not at all—from the arrival once, twice, or several times a day of some separated-out bran in the colon. Instead it will come from intact dietary fiber still in place where it belongs in foods, intimately associated with those foods, helping to produce satiety, helping to prevent excessive absorption of starches and sugars and possibly cholesterol in the diet, helping to prevent excessively rapid absorption that may disturb the proper secretion of insulin by the pancreas, and helping in many other ways.

Example of a High Fiber Meal Pattern †

BREAKFAST

Oatmeal, shredded wheat, or bran cereal, with milk and chopped fruit
Egg, bacon, tomatoes, or mushrooms

---

* In his advice to patients with constipation or diverticular disease who need to use bran, Dr. Painter suggests, as noted before, that they take one to two teaspoonfuls three times a day for two weeks and note its effects on the stools. "If the stools do not become softer," he adds, "the amount of bran should be increased even up to several tablespoonfuls a day until the motions are passed once a day, or better still twice, without straining. The ideal stool is formed and is of the diameter of the middle finger. Bran may cause flatulence for two or three weeks, but this soon clears up."

† Adapted from the United Bristol Hospitals *High Fibre Diet.*

Whole-meal bread (toasted if preferred) and butter
Coffee or tea without sugar

MIDMORNING
Coffee or tea without sugar

LUNCH
Meat, fish, eggs, or cheese
Vegetables
Potatoes
OR
Whole-meal bread sandwich, with cold meat, tuna fish, eggs, or cheese
Salad of tomatoes, cucumber, watercress, etc., or the same vegetables included in sandwich
Fresh or stewed fruit without sugar

MIDAFTERNOON
Coffee or tea without sugar
Nuts or dried fruit or whole-meal bread and butter

DINNER
Homemade vegetable soup
Meat, fish, cheese, or eggs
Vegetables—cooked or raw
Potatoes or whole-meal bread and butter
Fresh or stewed fruit without sugar

BEDTIME
Fresh fruit
Hot or cold milk

Example of a Very High Fiber Meal Pattern *

If you are troubled with constipation or another problem for which bran supplement may be indicated, your physician may suggest a meal pattern such as this:

BREAKFAST
Oatmeal, shredded wheat, or bran cereal, with milk plus dose of bran
Egg, bacon, ham, tomatoes
Whole-meal bread (toasted if preferred) and butter
Coarse marmalade
Coffee or tea without sugar

---

* Adapted from the United Bristol Hospitals *High Fibre Diet*.

MIDMORNING
Coffee or tea without sugar

LUNCH
Vegetable soup and dose of bran
Meat, fish, eggs, or cheese
Large serving of cooked vegetables
Potatoes, boiled or baked in their skins
OR
Whole-meal bread sandwich, with cold meat, tuna fish, eggs, or cheese
Salad of tomatoes, cucumber, watercress, etc., or the same vegetables included in sandwich
Fresh or stewed fruit without sugar

MIDAFTERNOON
Coffee or tea without sugar

DINNER
Meat, fish, cheese, or eggs
Large serving mixed raw vegetables, as a salad, with dose of bran
OR large serving cooked vegetables and dose of bran
Whole-meal bread and butter
OR potatoes, boiled or baked in their skins
Fresh fruit or pudding made with fruits or nuts

BEDTIME
Fresh fruit
Hot or cold milk

BRAN DOSAGE: 1 to 2 teaspoonfuls at a time—increased if necessary until a soft formed stool is passed without straining.

Some Ways of Taking Bran If Necessary*

1. You may try to take it dry but washed down with a glass of water, fruit juice, or other liquid, or you can mix it in with any of these liquids.
2. Mixed with breakfast cereal.
3. In soup.
4. In sauces, puddings, stewed fruit.
5. Added to whole-meal flour and used in baking. For each 4 cups unsifted whole-meal flour used, add ⅓ to ⅔ cup bran.

---

* Adapted from the United Bristol Hospitals *High Fibre Diet.*

Appendix: A previous safari (The Burkitt lymphoma)*

FROM the response to his 1,200 leaflets illustrated with photographs of children (p. 19), Burkitt was able to determine that the children's tumor appeared to be common in a belt across equatorial Africa from Kenya to Mozambique.

It was then that Burkitt, eager to go look at the situation and discover as much as possible about the disease and its predilections, set off with his two missionary friends in a station wagon on their 10,000-mile safari that lasted 10 weeks and included visits to 57 hospitals in 12 countries.

Conferences were held at the hospitals with doctors, nurses, and medical assistants. The prime purpose of the safari was not simply to visit hospitals reporting the tumor, but to discover where each patient was living when the tumor first appeared.

Burkitt got information—"Yes, we have seen a number of cases and they all came from this valley a few miles away"—or, another area twenty or forty miles away.

Then one day, as the three men drove along in the station wagon, discussing their findings, the realization came that altitude was a barrier to the tumor. Near the equator, no cases occurred above 5,000 feet; farther away from the equator, in Malawi, no

---

* For readers who are interested in a far more complete and very well-written account of the Burkitt lymphoma story, I recommend *Mr. Burkitt and Africa* by Bernard Glemser (New York: The World Publishing Company, 1970).

cases occurred above 3,000 feet; still farther away, in Swaziland, no cases occurred above 1,000 feet.

Why altitude? Burkitt pondered this upon completing the survey, and then with the very valuable help of a colleague, Professor A. J. Haddow, director of the East African Virus Research Institute, he found an explanation. The altitude barrier was really a temperature barrier. When altitudes were checked against climate patterns, it became apparent that wherever the temperature commonly fell below 60° F, children were unlikely to develop the tumor.

Still curious, Burkitt set out for West Africa after mailing his leaflets to mission and government hospitals there. In three weeks in West Africa he determined that the tumor was common in southern Nigeria but rare around Kano, 500 miles from Lagos. In Ghana the tumor could be found everywhere but around Accra on the coast.

Now it became apparent that rainfall was the critical factor. In southern Nigeria and Ghana annual rainfall ranges from 200 to 400 inches, but in Kano, close to the Sahara desert, no more than 10 to 20 inches fell a year, while Accra, too, is the driest part of the African coast.

Why were temperatures and rainfall critical factors? Burkitt went on another safari.

Rwanda, about the size of Maryland and the most densely populated African country, is southwest of Uganda, a high plateau with many mountains and lakes. Rwanda is famous for both its giant Batusi (or Watusi), some of whom are more than 7½ feet tall, and its Batwa, pygmies most of whom are 4 to 5 feet tall.

In Rwanda Burkitt found no evidence of the tumor at all. It had been seen in no hospitals in this country of high altitude.

But in Bujumbura, capital of Burundi, south of Rwanda, with an altitude of only 2,625 feet and a hot and humid climate, the tumor occurred.

Back in his office now, Burkitt had a tumor map, dotted with pins, showing where, from the evidence gathered in East and West Africa, Rwanda, and Bujumbura, the malignancy was common.

Professor Haddow now found that if chalk were rubbed all over a map of Africa and then wiped off from only those areas where rainfall was below 30 inches annually and temperatures fell below 60° F, what was left was a virtual duplicate of the tumor map.

And when Haddow considered what other possible map of Africa would have a similar pattern, it proved to be an insect map.

It was only a suspicion—that the tumor might be related to some insect. But in 1959 came an outbreak of a disease called o'nyong n'yong fever which, though rarely fatal, causes intense suffering, making its victims feel as if all their bones are broken.

The disease, starting in northwest Uganda, raged across northern Uganda, affecting 98 percent of the population. "But when it reached an altitude of 5,000 feet," Burkitt noted, "it stopped. It went around Lake Victoria. It went into part of southern Uganda. It went into Tanganyika. And everywhere it seemed to stop at about the same level as the tumor."

The fever is caused by a virus carried by a mosquito.

Circumstantial evidence is hardly conclusive, but the circumstantial evidence that Burkitt's lymphoma might be caused by a virus carried by mosquitoes was enough to arouse interest among scientists all over the world.

For many years cancer researchers, seeking causes of various forms of cancer, had considered that viruses might be among them. As early as 1908 investigators of leukemia had transmitted the disease from one chicken to another by injecting fluid obtained after filtering blood and tissue of an affected chicken and injecting it into a healthy chicken. The fluid was free of leukemic cells. And it was thought that the leukemia was induced by an infectious agent that must be a virus.

In 1951 investigators again were able to induce leukemia, this time in newborn mice, with a cell-free fluid obtained from leukemic mice, and the experimental conditions were such that the infectious agent could only be a virus.

Still other experiments in animals had pointed to a virus as a possible cause of leukemia. But what happens in animals does not necessarily apply to humans.

Burkitt's work gave new support to the virus theory. If a virus seemed to be involved in the lymphoma of African children—the lymphoma was later reported from many countries including Brazil, Columbia, New Guinea, India, England, Canada, Sweden, Japan, Thailand, and the United States—it could well be that a virus, even if not the same one, might be responsible for some forms of human leukemia and possibly other human cancers. And since many diseases caused by viruses can be avoided by vaccines, perhaps so might a proved virus-caused malignant disease.

Having determined that it was the lymphoma (now being named after him) that really had been the tumor in many malignancies formerly named according to the organ or structure most obviously involved—retinoblastoma when in the eye; granulosa cell tumor when in the ovary; neuroblastoma when in the adrenals; sarcoma when in the jaw—all of them treated surgically if at all and with no known survivors, Burkitt now set about trying to find a means of treatment other than surgery.

His earliest work—in conjunction with enthusiastic collaborators, some of them sent from Memorial Sloan-Kettering Cancer Center in New York—resulted in the first occasionally curative treatment employing large doses of a drug called methotrexate. Some of the patients originally given four to five days of methotrexate therapy in the very early sixties are still alive and considered cured.

Subsequently, Burkitt treated a series of patients with vincristine sulfate and a larger series with cyclophosphamide. The latter was considered to be the most effective and at the same time relatively inexpensive. It was given in a single injection, repeated once or twice at intervals of ten to fourteen days.

By 1966, when Burkitt left Africa, all early jaw lesions were showing total clinical remission after chemotherapy, and the long-term survival for tumors limited to the jaws was estimated at over 40 percent.

In that same year Dr. Joseph H. Burchenal of Sloan-Kettering and president of the American Association for Cancer Research gave a presidential address to the association and called it "Burkitt's tumor as a stalking horse for leukemia."

Burchenal noted that "the Oxford Dictionary defines a 'stalking-horse' as 'a horse trained to allow a fowler to conceal himself behind it or under its coverings in order to get within easy range of the game without alarming it.'" Thus, the title and its definition are meant to suggest that a careful study of Burkitt's tumor may provide a useful approach to the eventual control of acute leukemia.

A Burkitt's Tumor Subcommittee of the Acute Leukemia Task Force was formed, leading to establishment of a Lymphoma Treatment Center in Kampala, as a joint effort of the U.S. National Cancer Institute and the Uganda government and to the successes of Dr. John Ziegler, a National Cancer Institute researcher who was sent to Uganda to direct the center. By 1972 Dr. Ziegler was reporting overall long-term survival for 67 percent of patients with Burkitt's lymphoma.

The growing success of chemotherapy for the lymphoma stimulated investigations that have led to increasingly successful use of drugs, often in remarkable combinations, in acute leukemia and other malignancies.

For his lymphoma work Denis Burkitt has received innumerable awards and honors in addition to the Lasker Award. He has been made a Fellow of the Royal Society in England, an Honorary Fellow of the Royal College of Surgeons, Ireland. He is the recipient of the Gold Medal of the Society of Apothecaries, London; the Gardner Award, Canada; the Paul Ehrlich Gold Medal, Germany; the Gold Medal of the Irish Hospitals and Universities; the DuVilliers Award of the American Leukemia Society; the Catherine Judd Award of Sloan-Kettering; the Harrison Prize of the Royal College of Medicine; and the Stuart Prize of the British Medical Association.

In 1966, when Burkitt felt that it would be more useful for him to return to England and take a post with the Medical Research Council, in which he could go on to explore the geographical and epidemiological aspects of other forms of cancer, he left further work on Burkitt's lymphoma in very capable hands.

"Gradually, and quite correctly, other people," he says, "were going into all sorts of aspects of the tumor in much better fashion than I could. Someone took over treatment who knew far more about it than I did. Others went into electromicroscopy, histochemistry, and the rest. There are now over 800 papers published on this tumor.

"The way I look upon it is that my role was making tracks through the bush. Then experts came in with bulldozers and tarmac and made it into a big highway."

Where does the lymphoma stand now?

"I think it stands," says Burkitt, "that a virus called the EB virus is a good bet. The evidence suggesting the virus is very, very strong.

"The geographical distribution we believe to be related to hyperendemic malaria because we have never found the tumor common where malaria is not hyperendemic, never found malaria hyperendemic where the tumor is not common. And in animals, malaria has been given experimentally and has produced solid lymphomas with viruses in them.

"I think the best bet at the moment is that intense malaria causes a depression of the immune system of the body so that liability to lymphoma increases.

"A tremendously exciting project is under way now under the auspices of the National Cancer Institute of the United States and the International Agency for Cancer Research. Blood has been taken from 40,000 children in an area of about 500 square miles in northwest Uganda and is being kept in cold storage in Lyons,

France. It is expected that within a period of perhaps five years, about thirty cases will develop among the children who had their blood taken. Then the stored blood samples can be compared with fresh samples of the blood of these thirty children to see whether or not there has been a conversion of EB negative to EB positive antibodies, which would be a test for the implication of the EB virus."

COMPOSITION OF FOODS, 100 GRAMS (3.5 OUNCES), EDIBLE[1] PORTION

[Numbers in parentheses denote values imputed—usually from another form of the food or from a similar food. Zero in parentheses indicates that the amount of a constituent probably is none or is too small to measure. Dashes denote lack of reliable data for a constituent believed to be present in measurable amount. Calculated values, as those based on a recipe, are not in parentheses.] Note that there will often be more fiber in a given weight of a dehydrated or dried food than in the same weight of the fresh food, since with the elimination of the water the concentration of the other ingredients, including fiber, increases. Source: *United States Department of Agriculture Handbook No. 8*

	Calories	FIBER[2] Grams
Abalone:		
Raw	98	0
Canned	80	0
Acerola (Barbados-cherry or West Indian cherry), raw, pulp and skin.	28	.4
Acerola juice, raw	23	.3
Albacore, raw	177	0
Ale. See Beverages: Beer		
Alewife:		
Raw	127	0
Canned, solids and liquid	141	0
Algae. See Seaweeds		
Alimentary pastes. See Macaroni, Noodles, Pastinas, Spaghetti.		
Almonds:		
Dried	598	2.6
Roasted and salted	627	2.6
Sugar-coated. See Candy		
Almond meal, partially defatted	408	2.3
Amaranth, raw	36	1.3
Anchovy, pickled, with and without added oil, not heavily salted.	176	0
Apples:		
Raw, commercial varieties:		
Not pared	58	1.0
Pared	54	.6
Canned. See Applesauce		
Dehydrated, sulfured:		
Uncooked	353	3.8
Cooked, with added sugar	76	.5

	Calories	FIBER Grams
Dried, sulfured:		
Uncooked	275	3.1
Cooked	78	.9
Frozen, sliced, sweetened, not thawed	93	.7
Apple brown betty	151	.5
Apple butter	186	1.1
Apple juice, canned or bottled	47	.1
Applesauce, canned:		
Unsweetened or artificially sweetened	41	.6
Sweetened	91	.5
Apricots:		
Raw	51	.6
Candied	338	.6
Canned, solids and liquid	66	.4
Dehydrated, sulfured, nugget-type and pieces:		
Uncooked	332	3.8
Cooked, fruit and liquid, sugar added	119	.9
Dried, sulfured:		
Uncooked	260	3.0
Cooked, fruit and liquid:		
Without added sugar	85	1.0
With added sugar	122	.9
Frozen, sweetened, not thawed	98	.6
Apricot nectar, canned (approx. 40% fruit)	57	.2
Artichokes, globe or French:		
Raw		2.4
Cooked, boiled, drained		2.4
Artichokes, Jerusalem. See Jerusalem-artichokes		
Asparagus:		
Raw spears	26	.7

1 Edible portions apply to such foods as bread, milk, and boneless meat, which are totally edible, and to fruits, vegetables, and any other foods from which inedible parts have been removed before the food is weighed.

2 For explanation of the difference between crude fiber and dietary fiber, see page 121.

	Calories	FIBER Grams
Cooked spears, boiled, drained	20	.7
Canned spears:		
Regular pack:		
Solids and liquid	18	.5
Drained solids	21	.8
Drained liquid	11	Trace
Frozen:		
Not thawed	23	.8
Cooked, boiled, drained	22	.8
Avocados, raw:		
All commercial varieties	167	1.6
Baby foods: strained and chopped (or junior) foods, unless otherwise specified		
Cereals, precooked, dry, and other cereal products:		
Barley, added nutrients	348	1.2
High protein, added nutrients	357	2.2
Mixed, added nutrients	368	1.1
Oatmeal, added nutrients	375	1.5
Rice, added nutrients	371	.5
Teething biscuit	378	.7
Wheat. See Farina		
Desserts, canned:		
Custard pudding, all flavors	100	.2
Fruit pudding with starch base, milk and/or egg (banana, orange, or pineapple).	96	.3
Dinners, canned:		
Cereal, vegetable, meat mixtures (approx. 2%–4% protein):		
Beef noodle dinner	48	.3
Cereal, egg yolk, and bacon	82	.1
Chicken noodle dinner	49	.1
Macaroni, tomatoes, meat, and cereal	67	.3
Split peas, vegetables, and ham or bacon	80	.2
Vegetables and bacon, with cereal	68	.4
Vegetables and beef, with cereal	56	.4
Vegetables and chicken, with cereal	52	.2
Vegetables and ham, with cereal	64	.3
Vegetables and lamb, with cereal	58	.3
Vegetables and liver, with cereal	47	.3
Vegetables and liver, with bacon and cereal	57	.3
Vegetables and turkey, with cereal	44	.2
Meat or poultry (approx. 6%–8% protein):		
Beef with vegetables	87	.2
Chicken with vegetables	100	.2
Turkey with vegetables	86	.5
Veal with vegetables	63	.2

	Calories	FIBER Grams
Fruits and fruit products, with or without thickening, canned:		
Applesauce	72	.5
Applesauce and apricots	86	.5
Bananas (with tapioca or cornstarch, added ascorbic acid), strained.	84	.1
Bananas and pineapple (with tapioca or cornstarch)	80	.1
Fruit dessert with tapioca (apricot, pineapple, and/or orange)	84	.2
Peaches	81	.5
Pears	66	1.0
Pears and pineapple	69	.9
Plums with tapioca, strained	94	.3
Prunes with tapioca	86	.3
Meats, poultry, and eggs; canned		(0)
Vegetables, canned		
Beans, green	22	.8
Beets, strained	37	.6
Carrots	29	.6
Mixed vegetables, including vegetable soup	37	.5
Peas, strained	54	.8
Spinach, creamed	43	.4
Squash	25	.8
Sweet potatoes	67	.5
Tomato soup, strained	54	.2
Bacon, cured	665	0
Baking powders	78-172	Trace
Bamboo shoots, raw	27	.7
Bananas:		
Raw:		
Common	85	.5
Red	90	.4
Dehydrated, or banana powder	340	2.0
Bananas, baking type. See Plantain		
Barbados-cherry. See Acerola		
Barbecue sauce	91	.6
Barley, pearled:		
Light	349	.5
Pot or Scotch	348	.9
Barracuda, Pacific, raw	113	0
Basella. See Vinespinach		
Bass		0
Beans, broad. See Broadbeans		
Beans, common, mature seeds, dry:		
White:		
Raw	340	4.3

	Calories	FIBER Grams
Cooked	118	1. 5
Canned, solids and liquid	122	1. 4
Red:		
Raw	343	4. 2
Cooked	118	1. 5
Canned, solids and liquid	90	. 9
Pinto, calico, and red Mexican, raw	349	4. 3
Other, including black, brown, and Bayo, raw	339	4. 4
Beans, hyacinth. See Hyacinth-beans		
Beans, lima:		
Immature seeds:		
Raw	123	1. 8
Cooked, boiled, drained	111	1. 8
Canned:		
Regular pack:		
Solids and liquid	71	1. 3
Drained solids	96	1. 8
Drained liquid	20	Trace
Frozen:		
Not thawed	122	1. 9
Cooked, boiled, drained	118	1. 9
Mature seeds, dry:		
Raw	345	4. 3
Cooked	138	1. 7
Bean flour, lima	343	2.
Beans, mung:		
Mature seeds, dry, raw	340	4. 4
Sprouted seeds:		
Uncooked	35	. 7
Cooked, boiled, drained	28	. 7
Beans, snap	32	1. 0
Bean sprouts. See Beans, mung, and Soybeans		
Beans and frankfurters, canned	144	1. 0
Beaver, cooked, roasted	248	0
Beechnuts	568	3. 7
Beef		0
Beer. See Beverages		
Beets, common, red:		
Raw	43	. 8
Cooked, boiled, drained	32	. 8
Canned:		
Regular pack:		
Solids and liquid	34	. 5
Drained solids	37	. 8
Drained liquid	26	Trace

	Calories	FIBER Grams
Beet greens, common:		
Raw	24	1. 3
Cooked, boiled, drained	18	1. 1
Beverages, alcoholic and carbonated nonalcoholic:		
Alcoholic		0
Carbonated, nonalcoholic		(0)
Biscuits, baking powder	369	. 2
Biscuit dough, commercial, with enriched flour:		
Chilled in cans	277	. 2
Frozen	327	. 1
Biscuit mix, with enriched flour, and biscuits baked from mix:		
Mix, dry form	424	. 3
Biscuits, made with milk	325	. 2
Blackberries, including dewberries, boysenberries and youngberries, **raw.**	58	4. 1
Blackberries, canned, solids and liquid: with or without artificial sweetener	40	2. 8
Blackberries, frozen. See Boysenberries		
Blackberry juice, canned, unsweetened	37	Trace
Blackeye peas. See Cowpeas		
Blackfish. See Tautog		
Blanc mange. See Puddings		
Blueberries:		
Raw	62	1. 5
Canned, solids and liquid:		
Water pack, with or without artificial sweetener	39	1. 0
Sirup pack, extra heavy	101	. 9
Frozen, not thawed:		
Unsweetened	55	1. 5
Sweetened	105	. 9
Bluefish		0
Bockwurst. See Sausage		
Bologna. See Sausage		
Bonito, including Atlantic, Pacific, and striped; raw	168	0
Boston brown bread	211	. 7
Bouillon cubes or powder	120	–
Boysenberries:		
Canned, water pack, solids and liquid, with or without artificial sweetener	36	1. 9
Frozen, not thawed:		
Unsweetened	48	2. 7
Sweetened	96	1. 8
Brains, all kinds (beef, calf, hog, sheep), raw	125	0

	Calories	FIBER *Grams*
Bran:		
Added sugar and malt extract	240	7. 8
Added sugar and defatted wheat germ	238	6. 5
Bran flakes (40% bran), added thiamine	303	3. 6
Bran flakes with raisins, added thiamine	287	3. 0
Braunschweiger. See Sausage		
Brazilnuts	654	3. 1
Breads:		
Cracked-wheat	263	. 5
French or vienna	290	. 2
Italian	276	. 2
Raisin	262	. 9
Rye:		
American (⅓ rye, ⅔ clear flour)	243	. 4
Pumpernickel	246	1. 1
Salt-rising	267	. 2
White	269	. 2
Whole-wheat	243	1. 6
See also Biscuits; Boston brown bread; Cornbread; Muffins; Rolls; Salt sticks		
Breadcrumbs, dry, grated	392	. 3
Bread pudding with raisins	187	. 1
Bread sticks (vienna). See Salt sticks		
Bread stuffing mix and stuffings prepared from mix:		
Mix, dry form	371	. 8
Stuffing:		
Dry, crumbly: prepared with water, table fat	358	. 4
Moist: prepared with water, egg, table fat	208	. 2
Breadfruit, raw	103	1. 2
Breakfast cereals. See Corn, Oats, Rice, Wheat, also Bran, Farina.		
Broadbeans, raw:		
Immature seeds	105	2. 2
Mature seeds, dry	338	6. 7
Broccoli:		
Raw spears	32	1. 5
Cooked spears, boiled, drained	26	1. 5
Frozen	29	1. 1
Brown betty. See Apple brown betty		
Brownies. See Cookies		
Brussels sprouts:		
Raw	45	1. 6
Cooked, boiled, drained	36	1. 6
Frozen	36	1. 2
Buckwheat:		
Whole-grain	335	9. 9

	Calories	FIBER *Grams*
Flour:		
Dark	333	1. 6
Light	347	. 5
Buckwheat pancake mix. See Pancake mix		
Buffalofish, raw	113	0
Bulgur (parboiled wheat):		
Dry, commercial, made from—		
Club wheat	359	1. 7
Hard red winter wheat	354	1. 7
White wheat	357	1. 3
Canned, made from hard red winter wheat:		
Unseasoned	168	. 8
Seasoned	182	. 8
Bullhead, black, raw	84	0
Butter	716	0
Butter oil or dehydrated butter	876	0
Butterfish		0
Buttermilk:		
Fluid, cultured (made from skim milk)	36	0
Dried	387	0
Butternuts	629	—
Cabbage:		
Common varieties (Danish, domestic, and pointed types):		
Raw	24	. 8
Cooked, boiled until tender, drained:		
Shredded, cooked in small amount of water	20	. 8
Wedges, cooked in large amount of water	18	. 8
Dehydrated	308	10. 3
Red, raw	31	1. 0
Savoy, raw	24	. 8
Cabbage, Chinese (also called celery cabbage or pet-sai), compact heading type, raw.	14	. 6
Cabbage, spoon (also called white mustard cabbage or pakchoy), nonheading green leaf type:		
Raw	16	. 6
Cooked, boiled, drained	14	. 6
Cabbage salad. See Coleslaw		
Cakes: Unenriched cake flour used unless otherwise specified.		
Baked from home recipes	385	0–. 3
Fruitcake, made with enriched flour:		
Dark	379	. 6
Light	389	. 7
Cake mixes and cakes baked from mixes	438	0–. 4
Cake icings	376	0–. 8

	Calories	FIBER *Grams*
Cake icing mixes and icings made from mixes	409	.6
Candied fruits. See Apricots, Cherries, Citron, Figs, Ginger root, Grapefruit peel, Lemon peel, Orange peel, Pear, Pineapple		
Candy:		
Butterscotch	397	0
Candy corn. See Fondant		
Caramels:		
Plain or chocolate	399	.2
Plain or chocolate, with nuts	428	.4
Chocolate-flavored roll	396	.2
Chocolate:		
Bittersweet	477	1.8
Semisweet	507	1.0
Sweet	528	.5
Chocolate, milk:		
Plain	520	.4
With almonds	532	.7
With peanuts	543	.9
Chocolate-coated:		
Almonds	569	1.5
Chocolate fudge	430	.2
Chocolate fudge, with nuts	452	.4
Coconut center	438	.6
Fondant	410	.1
Fudge, caramel, and peanuts	433	.4
Fudge, peanuts, and caramel	459	.7
Honeycombed hard candy, with peanut butter	463	.4
Nougat and caramel	416	.2
Peanuts	561	1.2
Raisins	425	.6
Vanilla creams	435	.1
Fondant	364	Trace
Fudge:		
Chocolate	400	.2
Chocolate, with nuts	426	.4
Vanilla	398	0
Vanilla, with nuts	424	.2
Gum drops, starch jelly pieces	347	0
Hard	386	0
Jelly beans	367	Trace
Marshmallows	319	0
Mints, uncoated. See Fondant		
Peanut bars	515	1.2
Peanut brittle (no added salt or soda)	421	.5

	Calories	FIBER *Grams*
Sugar-coated:		
Almonds	456	.9
Chocolate discs	466	.3
Cantaloupes. See Muskmelons		
Cape-gooseberries. See Groundcherries		
Capicola. See Sausage, cold cuts, and luncheon meats		
Carambola, raw	35	.9
Caribou. See Reindeer		
Carissa (natalplum) raw	70	.9
Carob flour (St. Johnsbread)	180	7.7
Carp, raw	115	0
Carrots:		
Raw	42	1.0
Cooked, boiled, drained	31	1.0
Canned:		
Regular pack:		
Solids and liquid	28	.6
Drained solids	30	.8
Drained liquid	22	Trace
Dehydrated	341	9.3
Casaba melon. See Muskmelons		
Cashew nuts	561	1.4
Catfish, freshwater, raw	103	0
Catsup. See Tomato catsup		
Cauliflower:		
Raw	27	1.0
Cooked, boiled, drained	22	1.0
Frozen	22	.8
Caviar, sturgeon:		
Granular	262	—
Pressed	316	—
Celeriac, root, raw	40	1.3
Celery, all, including green and yellow varieties:		
Raw	17	.6
Cooked, boiled, drained	14	.6
Cereals, breakfast. See Corn, Oats, Rice, Wheat, also Bran, Farina		
Cervelat. See Sausage		
Chard, Swiss:		
Raw	25	0.8
Cooked, boiled, drained	18	.7
Charlotte russe, with ladyfingers, whipped-cream filling.	286	Trace

	Calories	FIBER Grams
Chayote, raw	28	.7
Cheeses, natural and processed; cheese foods; cheese spreads		0
Cheese fondue, from home recipe	265	Trace
Cheese souffle, from home recipe	218	Trace
Cheese straws	453	.1
Cherimoya, raw	94	2.2
Cherries	58	.1–.5
Cherries, maraschino, bottled, solids and liquid	116	.3
Chervil, raw	57	–
Chestnuts:		
Fresh	194	1.1
Dried	377	2.5
Chestnut flour	362	2.0
Chewing gum	317	–
Chicken:		
All classes		0
Chickpeas or garbanzos, mature seeds, dry, raw	360	5.0
Chicory, Witloof (also called French or Belgian endive), bleached head (forced), raw.	15	–
Chicory greens, raw	20	.8
Chili con carne, canned:		
With beans	133	.6
Without beans	200	.2
Chili powder. See Peppers		
Chili sauce. See Peppers; Tomatoes		
Chives, raw	28	1.1
Chocolate:		
Bitter or baking	505	2.5
Bittersweet. See Candy		
Chocolate sirup:		
Thin type	245	.6
Fudge type	330	.4
Chop suey, with meat:		
Cooked, from home recipe	120	.5
Canned	62	.8
Chow mein, chicken (without noodles):		
Cooked, from home recipe	102	.3
Canned	38	.3
Chub, raw	145	0
Cider. See Apple juice		
Cisco. See Lake herring		
Citron, candied	314	1.4
Clams		–
Cocoa and chocolate-flavored beverage powders:		
Cocoa powder with nonfat dry milk	359	.5

	Calories	FIBER Grams
Cocoa powder without milk	347	1.0
Mix for hot chocolate	392	.8
Cocoa, dry powder:		
High-fat or breakfast	299	4.3
Low-fat	187	5.8
Coconut cream (liquid expressed from grated coconut meat).	334	–
Coconut meat	346	4.0
Coconut milk (liquid expressed from mixture of grated coconut meat and water).		0
Coconut water (liquid from coconuts)	22	Trace
Cod		0
Coffee, instant, water-soluble solids:		
Dry powder	129	Trace
Beverage	1	Trace
Cola or coke. See Beverages		
Coleslaw	129	.7
Collards	45	1.2
Cookies:		
Assorted, packaged, commercial	480	.1
Brownies with nuts:		
Baked from home recipe, enriched flour	485	.7
Frozen, with chocolate icing, commercial	419	.6
Butter, thin, rich	457	.1
Chocolate	445	.3
Chocolate chip:		
Baked from home recipe, enriched flour	516	.4
Commercial type	471	.4
Coconut bars	494	.6
Fig bars	358	1.7
Gingersnaps	420	.1
Ladyfingers	360	.1
Macaroons	475	2.1
Marshmallow	409	.3
Molasses	422	.1
Oatmeal with raisins	451	.4
Peanut	473	.8
Raisin	379	.9
Sandwich type	495	.1
Shortbread	498	.2
Sugar, soft, thick, with enriched flour, home recipe	444	.1
Sugar wafers	485	.1
Vanilla wafers	462	.1

	Calories	FIBER Grams
Cooky mixes and cookies baked from mixes:		
Brownie, with enriched flour:		
Complete mix:		
Dry form	419	.5
Brownies, made with water, nuts	403	.7
Incomplete mix:		
Dry form	442	.5
Brownies, made with egg, water, nuts	428	.6
Plain, with unenriched flour:		
Mix, dry form	493	.1
Cookies, made with egg, water	493	.1
Cookies, made with milk	490	.1
Cooky dough, plain, chilled in roll:		
Unbaked	449	.1
Baked	496	.1
Cooking oil. See Oils		
Corn, field, whole-grain, raw	348	2.0
Corn, sweet:		
Raw, white and yellow	96	.7
Cooked, boiled, drained, white and yellow:		
Kernels, cut off cob before cooking	83	.7
Kernels, cooked on cob	**91**	**.7**
Canned:		
Regular pack:		
Cream style, white and yellow:		
Solids and liquid	**82**	**.5**
Whole kernel:		
Vacuum pack; yellow:		
Solids and liquid	**83**	**.8**
Wet pack, white and yellow:		
Solids and liquid	**66**	**.6**
Drained solids	**84**	**.8**
Drained liquid	**26**	**Trace**
Special dietary pack (low-sodium):		
Cream style, white and yellow:		
Solids and liquid	**82**	**.3**
Whole kernel, wet pack, white and yellow:		
Solids and liquid	**57**	**.5**
Drained solids	**76**	**.7**
Drained liquid	**17**	**Trace**
Frozen:		
Kernels, cut off cob:		
Not thawed	**82**	**.5**
Cooked, boiled, drained	**79**	**.5**
Kernels, on cob:		
Not thawed	**98**	**.7**

	Calories	FIBER Grams
Cooked, boiled, drained	94	.7
Corn flour	**368**	**.7**
Corn fritters	**377**	**.5**
Corn grits, degermed:		
Dry form	**362**	**.4**
Cooked	**51**	**.1**
Corn muffins. See Muffins, corn		
Corn oil. See Oils		
Corn products used mainly as ready-to-eat breakfast cereals:		
Corn flakes:		
Added nutrients	**386**	**.7**
Corn:	**386**	**.4**
puffed:		
Added nutrients	**399**	**.4**
Presweetened:		
Added nutrients	**379**	**.3**
Cocoa-flavored, added nutrients	**390**	**.5**
Fruit-flavored, added nutrients	**395**	**.3**
Corn, shredded, added nutrients	**389**	**.6**
Corn, rice, and wheat flakes, mixed, added nutrients	**389**	**1.2**
Corn, flaked, with protein concentrate (casein) and other added nutrients.	**378**	**.2**
Corn pudding	**104**	**.5**
Corn sirup. See Sirup, table blends		
Cornbread, baked from home recipes:		
Cornbread, southern style, made with—		
Whole-ground cornmeal	**207**	**.5**
Degermed cornmeal, enriched	**224**	**.2**
Johnnycake (northern style cornbread), made with enriched, yellow degermed cornmeal.	**267**	**.3**
Corn pone, made with white, whole-ground cornmeal	**204**	**.8**
Spoonbread, made with white whole-ground cornmeal.	**195**	**.3**
See also Muffins, corn		
Cornbread mix and cornbread baked from mix:		
Mix, dry form	432	0.3
Cornbread, made with egg, milk	233	.2
Cornmeal, white or yellow:		
Whole-ground, unbolted	355	1.6
Bolted (nearly whole-grain)	362	1.0
Degermed:		
Dry form	364	.6
Cooked	50	.1
Self-rising:		
Whole-ground	347	.9

	Calories	FIBER *Grams*
Degermed	348	.5
Cornsalad, raw	21	.8
Cornstarch	362	.1
Cottage pudding. See Cakes		
Cottonseed flour	356	2.0
Cottonseed oil. See Oils		
Cowpeas, including blackeye peas:		
Immature seeds:		
Raw	127	1.8
Cooked, boiled, drained	108	1.8
Canned, solids and liquid	70	.7
Mature seeds, dry:		
Raw	343	4.4
Cooked	76	1.0
Crab, including blue, Dungeness, rock and king:		
Cooked, steamed	93	–
Crab, canned	101	–
Crab, deviled	188	–
Crab imperial	147	–
Crabapples, raw	68	.6
Crackers:		
Animal	429	.1
Butter	458	.3
Cheese	479	.2
Graham:		
Chocolate-coated	475	.8
Plain	384	1.1
Sugar-honey coated	411	.8
Saltines	433	.4
Sandwich type, peanut-cheese	491	.5
Soda	439	.2
Whole-wheat	403	2.4
Cracker meal. See Crackers, soda		
Cranberries:		
Raw	46	1.4
Dehydrated, uncooked	368	8.7
Cranberry juice cocktail, bottled (approx. 33% cranberry juice).	65	Trace
Cranberry sauce, sweetened:		
Canned, strained	146	.2
Home-prepared, unstrained	178	.7
Cranberry-orange relish, uncooked	178	–
Crappie, white, raw	79	0
Crayfish, freshwater; and spiny lobster; raw	72	–
Cream		0
Cream substitutes	508	0
Cream puffs with custard filling	233	Trace

	Calories	FIBER *Grams*
Cress, garden:		
Raw	32	1.1
Cooked, boiled, drained, cooked	23	.9
Croaker, Atlantic:		
Raw	96	0
Cooked, baked	133	0
Croaker, white, raw	84	0
Croaker, yellowfin, raw	89	0
Cucumbers, raw:		
Not pared	15	.6
Pared	14	.3
Cucumber pickles. See Pickles		
Currants, raw:		
Black, European	54	2.4
Red and white	50	3.4
Cusk:		
Raw	75	0
Cooked, steamed	106	0
Custard, baked	115	0
Custard, frozen. See Ice cream		
Custard dessert mix. See Pudding mixes		
Custardapple, bullocksheart, raw	101	3.4
Daikon. See Radishes, oriental		
Dandelion greens:		
Raw	45	1.6
Cooked, boiled, drained	33	1.3
Danish pastry. See Rolls and buns		
Dasheens. See Taros		
Dates, domestic, natural and dry	274	2.3
Deviled ham. See Sausage		
Dewberries. See Blackberries		
Doughnuts:		
Cake type	391	.1
Yeast-leavened	414	.2
Duck	326	0
Eclairs with custard filling and chocolate icing	239	Trace
Eel, American, raw	233	0
Eel, smoked	330	0
Eggs		0
Eggplant:		
Raw	25	.9
Cooked, boiled, drained	19	.9
Elderberries, raw	72	7.0
Endive (curly endive and escarole), raw	20	.9
Escarole, raw. See Endive		
Eulachon (smelt), raw	118	0
Farina	371	.4

	Calories	FIBER *Grams*
Fats, cooking (vegetable fat)	884	0
Fennel, common, leaves, raw	28	.5
Figs:		
Raw	80	1.2
Dried, uncooked	**274**	**5.6**
Filberts (hazelnuts)	634	3.0
Finnan haddie (smoked haddock)	103	0
Fish. See individual kinds; Cod, etc.		
Flatfishes (flounders, soles, and sanddabs), raw	79	0
Flounder, cooked, baked	202	0
Flour. See Corn, Rice, Rye, Soya, Wheat		
Frankfurters. See Sausage		
Frog legs, raw	73	0
Frostings. See Cake icings		
Frozen custard. See Ice cream		
Fruit cocktail, canned, solids and liquid	60	.4
Fruit salad, canned, solids and liquid	59	.5
Garbanzos. See Chickpeas		
Garlic, cloves, raw	137	1.5
Gelatin	335	0
Gin. See Beverages		
Ginger ale. See Beverages		
Gingerbread. See Cakes		
Ginger root, crystallized (candied)	340	.7
Ginger root, fresh	49	1.1
Gizzard		0
Gizzard shad. See Shad, gizzard		
Gluten flour. See Wheat flours		
Goat milk. See Milk, goat		
Goose		0
Gooseberries:		
Raw	39	1.9
Canned, solids and liquid	90	1.3
Gourd, dishcloth. See Towelgourd		
Granadilla, purple (passionfruit) pulp and seeds, raw	90	—
Grapefruit	41	.2
Grapefruit peel, candied	316	2.3
Grapes	69	.6
Grapejuice	77	Trace
Griddlecakes. See Pancakes		
Grits. See Corn grits		
Groundcherries (poha or cape-gooseberries), raw	53	2.8
Grouper, including red, black, and speckled hind; raw	87	0
Guavas, whole, raw:		
Common	62	5.6

	Calories	FIBER *Grams*
Strawberry	65	6.4
Guinea hen	156	0
Haddock		0
Hake	74	0
Halibut		0
Ham. See Pork		
Ham croquette	251	.1
Hamburger. See Beef		
Haws, scarlet, flesh and skin, raw	87	2.1
Hazelnuts. See Filberts		
Headcheese. See Sausage		
Heart		0
Herring		0
Hickorynuts	673	1.9
Hominy grits, dry. See Corn grits		
Honey, strained or extracted	304	—
Honeydew melon. See Muskmelons		
Horseradish:		
Raw	87	2.4
Prepared	38	.9
Hyacinth-beans, raw:		
Young pods	35	1.8
Mature seeds, dry	338	6.9
Ice cream and frozen custard		0
Ice cream cones	377	.2
Ice milk	152	0
Ices, water, lime	78	Trace
Icings and icing mixes. See Cake icings		
Inconnu (sheefish), raw	146	0
Jack mackerel, raw	143	0
Jackfruit, raw	98	1.0
Jams and preserves	272	1.0
Jellies	273	0
Jerusalem artichoke, raw	50	.8
Jujube, common (Chinese date):		
Raw	105	1.4
Dried	287	3.0
Kale:		
Leaves, without stems, midribs	53	—
Leaves, including stems	38	1.3
Kidneys		0
Kingfish; southern, gulf, and northern (whiting); raw.	105	0
Knockwurst. See Sausage		

	Calories	FIBER Grams
Kohlrabi, thickened bulb-like stems:		
Raw	29	1.0
Cooked, boiled, drained	24	1.0
Kumquats, raw	65	3.7
Ladyfingers. See Cookies		
Lake herring (cisco), raw		0
Lake trout, raw		0
Lake trout		0
Lamb		0
Lambsquarters:		
Raw	43	2.1
Cooked, boiled, drained	32	1.8
Lard	902	0
Leeks, bulb and lower leaf portion, raw	52	1.3
Lemons, raw:		
Peeled fruit	27	0.4
Fruit, including peel	20	—
Lemon juice	25	Trace
Lemon peel:		
Raw	—	—
Candied	316	2.3
Lemonade concentrate, frozen:		
Undiluted	195	.1
Diluted with 4⅓ parts water, by volume	44	Trace
Lentils, mature seeds, dry:		
Whole:		
Raw	340	3.9
Cooked	106	1.2
Split, without seed coat, raw	345	1.7
Lettuce, raw:		
Butterhead varieties such as Boston types and Bibb	14	.5
Cos, or romaine, such as Dark Green and White Paris.	18	.7
Crisphead varieties such as Iceberg, New York, and Great Lakes strains.	13	.5
Looseleaf, or bunching varieties, such as Grand Rapids, Salad Bowl, Simpson.	18	.7
Lima beans. See Beans, lima		
Limes, acid type, raw	28	.5
Lime juice:		
Raw	26	Trace
Canned or bottled, unsweetened	26	Trace
Limeade concentrate, frozen:		
Undiluted	187	Trace
Diluted with 4⅓ parts water, by volume	41	Trace
Lingcod, raw	84	0

	Calories	FIBER Grams
Liver		0
Liver paste. See Pâté de foie gras		
Liver sausage or liverwurst. See Sausage		
Lobster, northern:		
Raw, whole	91	—
Canned or cooked	95	—
Lobster Newburg	194	—
Lobster salad	110	—
Lobster paste. See Shrimp or lobster paste, canned		
Lobster, spiny. See Crayfish		
Loganberries:		
Raw	62	3.0
Canned, solids and liquid:		
Water pack, with or without artificial sweetener	40	2.0
Juice pack	54	2.1
Sirup pack	70	2.0
Longans:		
Raw	61	.4
Dried	286	2.0
Loquats, raw	48	.5
Luncheon meat. See Sausage		
Lungs		0
Lychees:		
Raw	64	.3
Dried	277	1.4
Macadamia nuts	691	2.5
Macaroni:		
Dry form	369	.3
Cooked, firm stage (8–10 min.)	148	.1
Cooked, tender stage (14–20 min.)	111	.1
Macaroni and cheese:		
Baked, made from home recipe	215	.1
Canned	95	.1
Mackerel		0
Malt, dry	368	5.7
Malt extract, dried	367	Trace
Mamey (mammeeapple), raw	51	1.0
Mandarin oranges. See Tangerines		
Mangos, raw	66	.9
Margarine	720	0
Marmalade, citrus	257	.4
Marmalade plums. See Sapotes		
Matai. See Waterchestnut		
Mayonnaise. See Salad dressings		
Meat loaf. See Sausage		
Meat. See Beef, Lamb, Pork, Veal.		

	Calories	FIBER Grams
Melons. See Muskmelons, and Watermelons		
Menhaden, Atlantic, canned, solids and liquid	172	0
Milk		0
Millet, proso (broomcorn, hogmillet), whole-grain	**327**	3.2
Mixed vegetables, frozen. See Vegetables		
Molasses		—
Mortadella. See Sausage		
Muffins, baked from home recipes:		
Plain, made with—		
Enriched flour	294	.1
Unenriched flour	294	.1
Other, made with enriched flour:		
Blueberry	281	.3
Bran	261	1.8
Corn, made with—		
Enriched degermed cornmeal	314	.2
Whole-ground cornmeal	288	.5
Muffin mixes, corn, and muffins baked from mixes:		
Mix, dry form, with enriched flour	417	.5
Muffins, made with egg, milk	324	.2
Mix, dry form, with cake flour, nonfat dry milk	409	.2
Muffins, made with egg, water	297	.1
Mullet, striped, **raw**	146	0
Mushrooms:		
Agaricus campestris, cultivated commercially:		
Raw	28	.8
Canned, solids and liquid	17	.6
Other edible species, **raw**	35	1.1
Muskellunge, raw	109	0
Muskmelons:		
Raw:		
Cantaloups, other netted varieties	30	.3
Casaba (Golden Beauty)	27	.5
Honeydew	33	.6
Muskrat, cooked, roasted	153	0
Mussels, raw		—
Mustard greens:		
Raw	31	1.1
Cooked, boiled, drained	23	.9
Mustard spinach (tendergreen):		
Raw	22	1.0
Cooked, boiled, drained	16	.8
Mustard, prepared:		
Brown	91	1.3
Yellow	75	1.0
Nectarines, raw	64	.4

	Calories	FIBER Grams
New Zealand spinach:		
Raw	19	.7
Cooked, boiled, drained	13	.6
Noodles, egg noodles:		
Dry form	388	.4
Cooked	125	.1
Noodles, chow mein, canned	489	—
Nuts. See individual kinds		
Oat products used mainly as hot breakfast cereals:		
Oat cereal with toasted wheat germ and soy grits:		
Dry form	382	3.5
Cooked	62	.6
Oat flakes, maple-flavored, instant-cooking:		
Dry form	384	.7
Cooked	69	.1
Oat granules, maple-flavored, quick-cooking:		
Dry form	383	1.1
Cooked	60	.2
Oat and wheat cereal:		
Dry form	364	1.5
Cooked	65	.3
Oatmeal or rolled oats:		
Dry form	390	1.2
Cooked	55	.2
Oat products used mainly as ready-to-eat breakfast cereals:		
Oats, shredded, with protein and other added nutrients.	379	1.8
Oats (with or without corn), puffed, added nutrients	397	1.1
Oats (with or without corn, wheat), puffed, added nutrients, sugar-covered.	396	.7
Oats (with soy flour and rice), flaked, added nutrients	397	.9
Ocean perch		0
Octopus, raw	73	0
Oils, salad or cooking	884	0
Okra	36	1.0
Oleomargarine. See Margarine		
Olives, pickled; canned or bottled:		
Green	116	1.3
Ripe	129	1.4
Ripe, salt-cured, oil-coated, Greek style	338	3.8
Omelet. See Eggs		
Onions, mature (dry):		
Raw	38	.6
Cooked, boiled, drained	29	.6
Dehydrated, flaked	350	4.4

	Calories	FIBER *Grams*
Onions, young green (bunching varieties), raw:		
Bulb and entire top	36	(1. 2)
Bulb and white portion of top	45	1. 0
Tops only (green portion)	27	1. 3
Onions, Welsh, raw	34	1. 0
Opossum, cooked, roasted	221	0
Oranges	49	. 5
Orange juice	45	. 1
Orange-cranberry relish. See Cranberry-orange		
Orange juice and apricot juice drink, canned (approx. 40% fruit juices).	50	. 2
Orange peel	–	–
Oysters		–
Pancakes, baked from home recipe	231	. 1
Pancake and waffle mixes and pancakes baked from mixes:		
Buckwheat and other cereal flours:		
Mix, dry form	328	1. 4
Pancakes, made with egg, milk	200	. 4
Pancreas,		
Beef		0
Papaws, common, North American type, raw	85	–
Papayas, raw	39	. 9
Parsley, common garden (plain) and curled-leaf varieties, raw.	44	1. 5
Parsnips:		
Raw	76	2. 0
Cooked, boiled, drained	66	2. 0
Passionfruit. See Granadilla		
Pastinas, enriched, dry form:		
Egg	383	. 3
Vegetable:		
Carrot	371	. 6
Spinach	368	. 5
Pâté de foie gras, canned	462	0
Peaches:		
Raw	38	. 6
Canned, solids and liquid		. 4
Dehydrated, sulfured, nugget-type and pieces:		
Uncooked	340	(4. 0)
Cooked, fruit and liquid, with added sugar	121	(. 9)
Peach nectar, canned (approx. 40% fruit)	48	. 1
Peanuts:		
Raw, with skins	564	2. 4
Raw, without skins	568	1. 9
Boiled	376	1. 8
Roasted, with skins	582	2. 7
Roasted and salted	585	2. 4
Peanut butter	581	1. 9
Peanut spread	601	1. 5
Peanut flour, defatted	371	2. 7
Pears:		
Raw, including skin	61	1. 4
Canned, solids and liquid	32	. 7
Dried, sulfured:		
Uncooked	268	6. 2
Cooked, fruit and liquid:		
Without added sugar	126	2. 9
With added sugar	151	2. 6
Pear nectar, canned (approx. 40% fruit)	52	. 3
Peas, edible-podded:		
Raw	53	1. 2
Cooked, boiled, drained	43	1. 2
Peas, green, immature:		
Raw	84	2. 0
Cooked, boiled, drained	71	2. 0
Canned:		
Regular pack:		
Solids and liquid	66	1. 5
Drained solids	88	2. 3
Drained liquid	26	Trace
Frozen:		
Not thawed	73	1. 9
Cooked, boiled, drained	68	1. 9
Peas, mature seeds, dry:		
Whole:		
Raw	340	4. 9
Split, without seed coat:		
Raw	348	1. 2
Cooked	115	. 4
Peas and carrots, frozen:		
Not thawed	55	1. 5
Cooked, boiled, drained	53	1. 5
Pecans	687	2. 3
Peppers, hot, chili:		
Immature, green:		
Raw pods, excluding seeds	37	1. 8
Canned:		
Pods, excluding seeds; solids and liquid	25	1. 2
Chili sauce	20	1. 0
Mature, red:		
Raw:		
Pods, including seeds	93	9. 0

	Calories	FIBER *Grams*
Pods, excluding seeds	65	2.3
Canned, chili sauce	21	1.7
Dried:		
Pods	321	26.2
Chili powder with added seasoning	340	22.2
Peppers, sweet, garden varieties:		
Immature, green:		
Raw	22	1.4
Cooked:		
Boiled, drained	18	1.4
Stuffed with beef and crumbs	170	.7
Mature, red, raw	31	1.7
Perch, white, raw	118	0
Perch, yellow, raw	91	0
Persimmons, raw:		
Japanese or kaki	77	1.6
Native	127	1.5
Pheasant		0
Pickerel, chain, raw	84	0
Pickles		.5
Pies:		
Baked, piecrust made with unenriched flour:		
Apple	256	.4
Banana custard	221	.2
Blackberry	243	1.9
Blueberry	242	.7
Boston cream. See Cakes		
Butterscotch	267	Trace
Cherry	261	.1
Chocolate chiffon	328	.2
Chocolate meringue	252	.2
Coconut custard	235	.2
Custard	218	Trace
Lemon chiffon	313	Trace
Lemon meringue	255	Trace
Mince	271	.4
Peach	255	.4
Pecan	418	.5
Pineapple	253	.2
Pineapple chiffon	288	.1
Pineapple custard	220	.1
Pumpkin	211	.5
Raisin	270	.3
Rhubarb	253	.6
Strawberry	198	.8
Sweetpotato	213	.2

	Calories	FIBER *Grams*
Pigeonpeas, raw:		
Immature seeds	117	3.3
Mature seeds, dry	342	7.0
Pigs' feet, pickled	199	0
Pike, blue, raw	90	0
Pike, northern, raw	88	0
Pike, walleye, raw	93	0
Pilinuts	669	2.7
Pimientos, canned, solids and liquid	27	.6
Pineapple:		
Raw	52	0.4
Candied	316	.8
Canned, solids and liquid:		
Water pack, all styles except crushed, with or without artificial sweetener.	39	.3
Juice pack, all styles	58	.3
Sirup pack, all styles:		
Light	59	.3
Heavy	74	.3
Extra heavy	90	.3
Frozen chunks, sweetened, not thawed	85	.3
Pineapple juice:		
Canned, unsweetened	55	.1
Frozen concentrate, unsweetened:		
Undiluted	179	.3
Diluted with 3 parts water, by volume	52	.1
Pineapple juice and grapefruit juice drink, canned (approx. 40% fruit juices).	54	Trace
Pineapple juice and orange juice drink, canned (approx. 40% fruit juices).	54	Trace
Pinenuts:		
Pignolias	552	.9
Piñon	635	1.1
Pistachionuts	594	1.9
Pitanga (Surinam-cherry), raw	51	.6
Pizza, with cheese:		
From home recipe, baked:		
With cheese topping	236	.3
With sausage topping	234	.3
Chilled:		
Partially baked	208	.3
Baked	245	.3
Frozen:		
Partially baked	229	.3
Baked	245	.3
Plantain (baking banana), raw	119	.4

	Calories	FIBER Grams
Plate dinners, frozen, commercial, unheated:		
Beef pot roast, whole oven-browned potatoes, peas, and corn.	106	.3
Chicken, fried; mashed potatoes; mixed vegetables (carrots, peas, corn, beans).	173	.4
Meat loaf with tomato sauce, mashed potatoes, and peas.	131	.3
Turkey, sliced; mashed potatoes; peas	112	.3
Plums:		
Raw:		
Damson	66	.4
Japanese and hybrid	48	.6
Prune-type	75	.4
Canned, solids and liquid:		
Greengage, water pack, with or without artificial sweetener.	33	.2
Purple (Italian prunes):		
Water pack, with or without artificial sweetener.	46	.3
Sirup pack:		
Light	63	.3
Heavy	83	.3
Extra heavy	102	.3
Poha. See Groundcherries		
Pokeberry (poke) **shoots:**		
Raw	23	—
Cooked, boiled, drained	20	—
Pollock:		
Raw	95	0
Cooked, creamed	128	—
Pomegranate pulp, raw	63	.2
Pompano, raw	166	0
Popcorn:		
Unpopped	362	2.1
Popped:		
Plain	386	2.2
Oil and salt added	456	1.7
Sugar-coated	383	1.1
Popovers, baked (from home recipe with enriched flour).	224	.1
Porgy and scup, raw	112	0
Pork		0
Potatoes:		
Raw	76	.5
Cooked:		
Baked in skin	93	.6
Boiled in skin	76	.5
Boiled, pared before cooking	65	.5
French-fried	274	1.0
Potato chips	568	(1.6)
Potato flour	351	1.6
Potato salad, from home recipe, made with—		
Cooked salad dressing, seasonings	99	.4
Mayonnaise and French dressing, hard-cooked eggs, seasonings.	145	.4
Potato sticks	544	1.5
Pretzels	390	.3
Pricklypears, raw	42	1.6
Prunes:		
Dehydrated, nugget-type and pieces:		
Uncooked	344	(2.2)
Cooked, fruit and liquid, with added sugar	180	(.8)
Dried, "softenized":		
Uncooked	255	1.6
Cooked (fruit and liquid):		
Without added sugar	119	.8
With added sugar	172	.6
Prune juice, canned or bottled	77	Trace
Prune whip	156	.6
Puddings with starch base, prepared from home recipe:		
Chocolate	148	.2
Vanilla (blanc mange)	111	Trace
See also Bread; Rennin products; Rice; Tapioca; Baby foods		
Pudding mixes and puddings made from mixes:		
With starch base:		
Mix, chocolate, regular, dry form	361	.6
Pudding made with milk, cooked	124	.1
Mix, chocolate, instant, dry form	357	.6
Pudding made with milk, without cooking	125	.1
With vegetable gum base:		
Mix, custard-dessert, dry form	384	Trace
Pudding made with milk, cooked	131	Trace
Pumpkin:		
Raw	26	1.1
Canned	33	1.3
Pumpkin and squash seed kernels, dry	553	1.9
Purslane leaves, including stems:		
Raw	21	.9
Cooked, boiled, drained	15	.8
Quail	168	0
Quinces, raw	57	1.7
Rabbit		0

	Calories	FIBER Grams
Raccoon, cooked, roasted	255	0
Radishes, raw:		
Common	17	.7
Oriental, including daikon (Japanese) and Chinese	19	.7
Raisins, natural (unbleached):		
Uncooked	289	.9
Cooked, fruit and liquid, added sugar	213	.4
Raja fish. See Skate		
Raspberries:		
Raw:		
Black	73	5.1
Red	57	3.0
Canned, solids and liquid, water pack, with or without artificial sweetener:		
Black	51	3.3
Red	35	2.6
Frozen, red, sweetened, not thawed	98	2.2
Red and gray snapper, raw	93	0
Redfish. See Ocean perch		
Redhorse, silver	98	0
Reindeer		0
Rennin products:		
Chocolate:		
Mix, dry form	387	.9
Dessert made with milk	102	.1
Rhubarb, raw	16	.7
Rice:		
Brown:		
Raw	360	.9
Cooked	119	.3
White (fully milled or polished):		
Enriched:		
Common commercial varieties, all types:		
Raw	363	.3
Cooked	109	.1
Long-grain:		
Parboiled:		
Dry form	369	.2
Cooked	106	.1
Precooked (instant):		
Dry form	374	.4
Ready-to-serve	109	.1
Unenriched:		
Common commercial varieties, all types:		
Raw	363	.3

	Calories	FIBER Grams
Cooked	109	.1
Glutinous (Mochi Gomi), raw	361	.3
Rice bran	276	11.5
Rice polish	265	2.4
Rice products used mainly as hot breakfast cereals:		
Rice, granulated, added nutrients:		
Dry form	383	.2
Cooked	50	**Trace**
Rice products used mainly as ready-to-eat breakfast cereals:		
Rice flakes, added nutrients	390	.6
Rice, puffed; added nutrients, without salt	399	.6
Rice, puffed or oven-popped, presweetened:		
Honey and added nutrients	388	.2
Honey or cocoa and added nutrients, including fat.	401	.4
Rice, shredded; added nutrients	392	.3
Rice, with protein concentrate, mainly—		
Casein, other added nutrients	382	.5
Wheat gluten, other added nutrients	386	.5
Rice pudding with raisins	146	.1
Rockfish		0
Roe		—
Rolls and buns:		
Baked from home recipe, with milk and enriched flour.		
Commercial:		
Ready-to-serve:		
Danish pastry	422	.1
Hard rolls	312	.2
Plain (pan rolls)	298	.2
Raisin rolls or buns	275	.9
Sweet rolls	316	.2
Whole-wheat rolls	257	1.6
Partially baked (brown-and-serve)	299	.2
Roll dough and rolls baked from dough:		
Dough, unraised, frozen	268	.2
Rolls, baked	311	.3
Roll mix and rolls baked from mix:		
Mix, dry form	393	.2
Rolls, made with water	299	.2
Root beer. See Beverages		
Roseapples, raw	56	1.1
Rum. See Beverages		
Rusk	419	.2

	Calories	FIBER Grams
Rutabagas:		
Raw	46	1. 1
Cooked, boiled, drained	35	1. 1
Rye:		
Whole-grain	334	2. 0
Flours:		
Light	357	. 4
Medium	350	1. 0
Dark	327	2. 4
Rye wafers, whole-grain	344	2. 2
Sablefish, raw	190	0
Safflower seed kernels, dry	615	–
Safflower seed meal, partially defatted	355	7. 4
Salad dressings, commercial:		
Blue and Roquefort cheese	504	. 1
French	410	. 3
Italian	552	Trace
Mayonnaise	718	Trace
Russian	494	. 3
Salad dressings, made from home recipe:		
French	632	. 1
Cooked	164	0
Salad oil. See Oils		
Salami. See Sausage		
Salmon		0
Salsify:		
Raw	13–82	1. 8
Cooked, boiled, drained	12–70	1. 8
Salt, table	0	0
Salt pork, raw	783	0
Salt sticks:		
Regular type	384	. 3
Vienna bread type	304	. 2
Sanddab. See Flatfishes		
Sandwich spread (with chopped pickle):		
Regular	379	. 4
Special dietary (low-calorie, approx. 5 Cal. per tsp.)	112	. 4
Sapodilla, raw	89	1. 4
Sapotes (marmalade plums), raw	125	1. 9
Sardines, Atlantic, canned in oil:		
Solids and liquid	311	–
Drained solids	203	–
Sausage, cold cuts, and luncheon meats		0
Scallops		–
Scrapple. See Sausage		
Scup. See Porgy		

	Calories	FIBER Grams
Seabass, white, raw	96	0
Seaweeds, raw:		
Agar	–	. 7
Dulse	–	1. 2
Irishmoss	–	2. 1
Kelp	–	6. 8
Laver	–	3. 5
Sesame seeds, dry:		
Whole	563	6. 3
Decorticated	582	2. 4
Shad		0
Shad, gizzard (gizzard shad), **raw**	200	0
Shallot bulbs, raw	72	. 7
Sheefish. See Inconnu		
Sheepshead, Atlantic, raw	113	0
Sherbet, orange	134	0
Shortbread. See Cookies		
Shrimp		–
Sirups		0
Siscowet. See Lake trout		
Skate (raja fish), raw	98	0
Smelt		0
Snail, raw	90	–
Snail, Giant African, raw	73	–
Snapper, red. See Red and gray snapper		
Soft drinks. See Beverages		
Sole. See Flatfishes		
Sorghum grain, all types	332	1. 7
Soups,		
commercial:		
Canned:		
Asparagus, cream of:		
Condensed	54	. 6
Prepared with equal volume of water	27	. 3
Prepared with equal volume of milk	60	. 3
Bean with pork:		
Condensed	134	1. 3
Prepared with equal volume of water	67	. 6
Beef broth, bouillon, and consomme:		
Condensed	26	. 1
Prepared with equal volume of water	13	Trace
Beef noodle:		
Condensed	57	. 1
Prepared with equal volume of water	28	Trace
Celery, cream of:		
Condensed	72	. 4

	Calories	FIBER *Grams*
Prepared with equal volume of water	36	.2
Prepared with equal volume of milk	69	.2
Chicken consomme:		
Condensed	18	Trace
Prepared with equal volume of water	9	Trace
Chicken, cream of:		
Condensed	79	.1
Prepared with equal volume of water	39	.1
Prepared with equal volume of milk	73	.1
Chicken gumbo:		
Condensed	46	.2
Prepared with equal volume of water	23	.1
Chicken noodle:		
Condensed	53	.1
Prepared with equal volume of water	26	.1
Chicken with rice:		
Condensed	39	.1
Prepared with equal volume of water	20	Trace
Chicken vegetable:		
Condensed	62	.3
Prepared with equal volume of water	31	.1
Clam chowder, Manhattan type (with tomatoes, without milk):		
Condensed	66	.3
Prepared with equal volume of water	33	.2
Minestrone:		
Condensed	87	.6
Prepared with equal volume of water	43	.3
Mushroom, cream of:		
Condensed	111	.2
Prepared with equal volume of water	56	.1
Prepared with equal volume of milk	88	.1
Onion:		
Condensed	54	.4
Prepared with equal volume of water	27	.2
Pea, green:		
Condensed	106	.9
Prepared with equal volume of water	53	.4
Prepared with equal volume of milk	85	.4
Pea, split:		
Condensed	118	.4
Prepared with equal volume of water	59	.2
Tomato:		
Condensed	72	.4
Prepared with equal volume of water	36	.2
Prepared with equal volume of milk	69	.2

	Calories	FIBER *Grams*
Turkey noodle:		
Condensed	65	.1
Prepared with equal volume of water	33	.1
Vegetable beef:		
Condensed	65	0.4
Prepared with equal volume of water	32	.2
Vegetable with beef broth:		
Condensed	64	.5
Prepared with equal volume of water	32	.3
Vegetarian vegetable:		
Condensed	64	.4
Prepared with equal volume of water	32	.2
Dehydrated:		
Beef noodle:		
Mix, dry form	387	.6
Prepared with 2 oz. mix in 3 cups water	28	Trace
Chicken noodle:		
Mix, dry form	383	.4
Prepared with 2 oz. mix in 4 cups water	22	Trace
Chicken rice:		
Mix, dry form	353	.2
Prepared with 1½ oz. mix in 3 cups water	20	Trace
Onion:		
Mix, dry form	349	1.8
Prepared with 1½ oz. mix in 4 cups water	15	.1
Pea, green:		
Mix, dry form	362	1.2
Prepared with 2 oz. mix in 3 cups water	50	.2
Tomato vegetable with noodles:		
Mix, dry form	348	1.5
Prepared with 2½ oz. mix in 4 cups water	27	.1
Frozen:		
Clam chowder, New England type (with milk, without tomatoes):		
Condensed	107	.2
Prepared with equal volume of water	54	.1
Prepared with equal volume of milk	86	.1
Pea, green, with ham:		
Condensed	113	1.4
Prepared with equal volume of water	57	.7
Potato, cream of:		
Condensed	87	.3
Prepared with equal volume of water	44	.2
Prepared with equal volume of milk	76	.2

	Calories	FIBER Grams
Shrimp, cream of:		
Condensed	133	.3
Prepared with equal volume of water	66	.2
Prepared with equal volume of milk	99	.2
Vegetable with beef:		
Condensed	70	.5
Prepared with equal volume of water	35	.2
Soursop, raw	65	1.1
Souse. See Sausage		
Soybeans:		
Immature seeds:		
Raw	134	1.4
Cooked, boiled, drained	118	1.4
Canned:		
Solids and liquid	75	.7
Drained solids	103	1.4
Mature seeds, dry:		
Raw	403	4.9
Cooked	130	1.6
Fermented products:		
Natto (soybeans)	167	3.2
Miso (cereal and soybeans)	171	2.3
Sprouted seeds:		
Raw	46	.8
Cooked, boiled, drained	38	.8
Soybean curd (tofu)	72	.1
Soybean flours	421	2.4
Soybean milk:		
Fluid	33	0
Powder	429	.2
Soybean milk products, sweetened:		
Liquid concentrate	126	.2
Powder	452	.5
Soybean protein	322	.4
Soybean proteinate	312	.6
Soy sauce	68	0
Spaghetti		.1–.3
Spanish mackerel, raw	177	0
Spanish rice, cooked from home recipe	87	.5
Spinach:		
Raw	26	.6
Cooked, boiled, drained	23	.6
Canned:		
Regular pack:		
Solids and liquid	19	.7
Drained solids	24	.9

	Calories	FIBER Grams
Drained liquid	6	Trace
Frozen	24	.8
Spinach, New Zealand. See New Zealand spinach		
Squash:		
Summer:		
All varieties	19	0.6
Winter:		
All varieties	50	1.4
Squid, raw		—
Starch. See Cornstarch		
St. Johnsbread. See Carob flour		
Stomach, pork, scalded	152	0
Strawberries:		
Raw	37	1.3
Canned, solids and liquid:		
Water pack, with or without artificial sweetener	22	.6
Frozen, sweetened, not thawed:		
Sliced	109	.8
Whole	92	.6
Sturgeon		0
Succotash (corn and lima beans), frozen:		
Not thawed	97	.9
Cooked, boiled, drained	93	.9
Suckers, including white and mullet suckers, raw	104	0
Sucker, carp, raw	111	0
Suet (beef kidney fat), raw	854	0
Sugars:		
Beet or cane:		
Brown	373	0
Granulated	385	0
Powdered	385	0
Dextrose:		
Anhydrous	366	0
Crystallized	335	0
Maple	348	—
Sugarapples (sweetsop), raw	94	1.7
Sunflower seed kernels, dry	560	3.8
Sunflower seed flour, partially defatted	339	4.6
Surinam-cherry. See Pitanga		
Swamp cabbage:		
Raw	29	1.1
Cooked, boiled, drained	21	.9
Sweetbreads (thymus)		0

	Calories	FIBER Grams
Sweetpotatoes:		
Raw:		
All commercial varieties	114	.7
Cooked, all:		
Baked in skin	141	.9
Boiled in skin	114	.7
Candied	168	.6
Canned:		
Liquid pack, solids and liquid:		
Regular pack in sirup	114	.6
Special dietary pack, without added sugar and salt.	46	.3
Vacuum or solid pack	108	1.0
Dehydrated flakes:		
Dry form	379	3.2
Prepared with water	95	.8
Sweetsop. See Sugarapples		
Swisschard. See Chard		
Swordfish		0
Tamarinds, raw	239	5.1
Tangelo juice, raw	41	Trace
Tangerines, raw (Dancy variety)	46	.5
Tangerine juice		(.1)
Tapioca, dry	352	.1
Tapioca desserts:		
Apple tapioca	117	.1
Tapioca cream pudding	134	0
Taros, raw:		
Corms and tubers	98	.8
Leaves and stems	40	1.4
Tartar sauce:		
Regular	531	0.3
Special dietary (low-calorie, approx. 10 Cal. per tsp.)	224	.3
Tautog (blackfish), raw	89	0
Tea, instant (water-soluble solids) carbohydrate added:		
Dry powder	294	.1
Beverage	2	Trace
Tendergreen. See Mustard spinach		
Terrapin (diamond back), raw	111	0
Thuringer. See Sausage		
Tilefish:		
Raw	79	0
Cooked, baked	138	0
Tomatoes, green, raw	24	.5

	Calories	FIBER Grams
Tomatoes, ripe:		
Raw	22	.5
Cooked, boiled	26	.6
Canned, solids and liquid:		
Regular pack	21	.4
Special dietary pack (low-sodium)	20	.4
Tomato catsup, bottled	106	.5
Tomato chili sauce, bottled	104	.7
Tomato juice:		
Canned or bottled:		
Regular pack	19	.2
Special dietary pack (low-sodium)	19	.2
Canned concentrate:		
Undiluted	76	.9
Diluted with 3 parts water, by volume	20	.2
Dehydrated (crystals):		
Dry form	303	3.1
Prepared with water (1 lb. yields approx. 1¾ gals.).	20	.2
Tomato juice cocktail, canned or bottled	21	.2
Tomato paste, canned	82	.9
Tomato puree, canned:		
Regular pack	39	.4
Special dietary pack (low-sodium)	39	.4
Tomcod, Atlantic, raw	77	0
Tongue		0
Towelgourd, raw	18	.5
Tripe, beef:		
Commercial	100	0
Trout. See Lake trout		
Tuna		0
Turnips:		
Raw	30	.9
Cooked, boiled, drained	23	.9
Turnip greens, leaves, including stems:		
Raw	28	.8
Cooked, boiled, drained, cooked in—		
Small amount of water, short time	20	.7
Large amount of water, long time	19	.7
Canned, solids and liquid	18	0.7
Frozen:		
Not thawed	23	1.0
Cooked, boiled, drained	23	1.0
Turtle, green:		
Raw	89	0

	Calories	FIBER *Grams*
Veal	**207**	**0**
Vegetable juice cocktail, canned	17	. 3
Vegetable main dishes, canned, principal ingredients:		
Peanuts and soya	237	. 9
Wheat protein	109	. 1
Wheat protein, nuts or peanuts	212	. 4
Wheat protein, vegetable oil	189	—
Wheat and soy protein	104	. 3
Wheat and soy protein, soy or other vegetable oil	150	. 6
Vegetables, mixed (carrots, corn, peas, green snap beans, lima beans), frozen:		
Not thawed	65	1. 2
Cooked, boiled, drained	64	1. 2
Vegetable-oyster. See Salsify		
Venison, lean meat only, raw	126	0
Vienna sausage. See Sausage		
Vinegar:		
Cider	14	—
Distilled	12	—
Vinespinach (basella), raw	19	. 7
Vodka. See Beverages		
Waffles:		
Baked from home recipe, made with—		
Enriched flour	279	. 1
Unenriched flour	279	. 1
Frozen, made with enriched flour	253	. 2
Waffle mixes and waffles baked from mixes:		
Mix, with enriched flour, dry form	458	. 2
Waffles, made with water	305	. 1
Mix, with unenriched flour, dry form	458	. 2
Waffles, made with water	305	. 1
Mix (pancake and waffle), with enriched flour, dry form.	356	. 4
Waffles, made with egg, milk	275	. 2
Mix (pancake and waffle), with unenriched flour, dry form.	356	. 4
Waffles, made with egg, milk	275	. 2
Walnuts:		
Black	628	1. 7
Persian or English	651	2. 1
Waterchestnut, Chinese (matai, waternut), raw	79	. 8
Watercress leaves including stems, raw	19	. 7
Water ice. See Ices, water		
Watermelon, raw	26	. 3
Waxgourd (Chinese preserving melon), raw	13	. 5

	Calories	FIBER *Grams*
Weakfish:		
Raw	121	0
Cooked, broiled	208	0
Welsh rarebit	179	0
West Indian Cherry. See Acerola		
Whale meat, raw	156	0
Wheat, whole-grain:		
Hard red spring	330	2. 3
Hard red winter	330	2. 3
Soft red winter	326	2. 3
White	335	1. 9
Durum	332	1. 8
Wheat flours:		
Whole (from hard wheats)	333	2. 3
80% extraction (from hard wheats)	365	. 5
Straight, hard wheat	365	. 4
Straight, soft wheat	364	. 4
Patent:		
All-purpose or family flour:		
Enriched	364	. 3
Unenriched	364	. 3
Bread flour:		
Enriched	365	. 3
Unenriched	365	. 3
Cake or pastry flour	364	. 2
Gluten flour (45% gluten, 55% patent flour)	378	. 4
Self-rising flour, enriched (anhydrous monocalcium phosphate used as a baking acid).	352	. 4
Wheat bran, crude, commercially milled	213	9. 1
Wheat germ, crude, commercially milled	363	2. 5
Wheat, parboiled. See Bulgur		
Wheat products used mainly as hot breakfast cereals:		
Wheat, rolled:		
Dry form	340	2. 2
Cooked	75	. 5
Wheat, whole-meal:		
Dry form	338	2. 2
Cooked	45	. 3
Wheat and malted barley cereal, toasted:		
Quick-cooking:		
Dry form	383	1. 5
Cooked	65	. 2
Instant-cooking:		
Dry form	382	1. 6
Cooked	80	. 3
Also see Farina		

	Calories	FIBER *Grams*
Wheat products used mainly as ready-to-eat breakfast cereals:		
Wheat bran. See Bran		
Wheat flakes, added nutrients	354	1. 6
Wheat germ, toasted	391	1. 7
Wheat, puffed:		
Added nutrients, without salt	363	2. 0
Added nutrients,[171] with sugar and honey	376	. 9
Wheat, shredded:		
Without salt or other added ingredients	354	2. 3
With malt, salt, and sugar added	366	2. 2
Wheat and malted barley flakes, nutrients added	392	1. 8
Wheat and malted barley granules, nutrients added	391	1. 5
Whey:		
Fluid	26	0
Dried	349	0
Whisky. See Beverages		
Whitefish		0

	Calories	FIBER *Grams*
White sauce		Trace
Whiting. See Kingfish		
Wild rice, raw	353	1. 0
Wine. See Beverages		
Wreckfish, raw	114	0
Yam, tuber, raw	101	. 9
Yambean, tuber, raw	55	. 7
Yeast:		
Baker's:		
Compressed	86	—
Dry (active)	282	—
Brewer's, debittered	283	1. 7
Torula	277	3. 3
Yellowtail (Pacific coast), **raw**	138	0
Yoghurt		0
Youngberries. See Blackberries		
Zwieback	423	. 3

High fiber recipes

The following recipes—which will also be used in their clinic—have been prepared especially for this book by the Bristol Royal Infirmary, Department of Dietetics. The department is responsible for the original diet recommendations endorsed by Dr. Burkitt and his colleagues found in Chapter 17.

Equivalents

1 cup flour	=	4 oz.
1 cup fat	=	8 oz.
1 cup soft bread crumbs	=	2 oz.
1 cup rice (uncooked)	=	6 oz.
1 cup mixed fruit	=	4 oz.
1 cup grated cheese	=	4 oz.
1 cup of nuts (chopped)	=	4 oz.
1 cup of coconut	=	2½ oz.
1 cup liquid	=	8 oz.

In these recipes we have eliminated refined carbohydrates—this has meant finding substitutes for regular wheat, corn flour, sugar, molasses, syrup, and honey (except in two bread and one pizza recipe where a nominal amount is used to hasten rising).

Regular wheat and corn flour have been replaced by whole-meal wheat flour, oats, or other whole-grain cereals. This is quite a simple substitution and does not affect the quality of the food.

The best substitutes for sugar, molasses, syrup, and honey are fresh, dried, or purėed fruits. Nuts, spices, and fresh cream can be used to add interest and variety, but inevitably the texture and taste of the final product is altered.

It may take a short time to adjust to the more subtle flavors of unrefined cookery. Also switching to an unrefined food intake will mean a lot more baking than you are used to, as most of the regular convenience foods are very refined, and therefore totally unsuitable. However, you will find great satisfaction in creating these unrefined dishes.

The majority of the recipes will serve four, except of course cakes and cookies and party foods, where the portions will depend on individual appetites or as otherwise noted.

Bran

By eating unrefined foods your fiber intake is greatly increased, but you can boost it even further by taking unprocessed bran. There are many ways of incorporating bran into your food.

You will find various suggestions throughout the recipe section. But some simpler ways are to stir bran into drinks, soups, and gravies, or to sprinkle it over stewed fruit, cooked vegetables, and breakfast cereals.

The following suggestions offer guidelines to unrefined cookery, but use your imagination to adapt these ideas and build up your own collection of favorite recipes. Soon you will find an exciting new experience in food.

Starters

Most popular starters will be suitable, especially the fruity ones, e.g., grapefruit, melon, avocado, etc. Try to use spices to add interest wherever possible and where you would regularly use sugar.

Listed below are some appetizers you might find useful:

1. Plain or spiced grapefruit. Try broiling fresh grapefruits cut in half and topped with cinnamon and ginger.
2. Chilled melon plain or with orange segments or other soft fruits.
3. Small pieces of meat and fish with a white or cheese sauce (see Sauces) and glazed with aspic jelly.
4. A selection of shellfish with mayonnaise (see Salads) and lemon wedges. Thin slices of whole-meal bread and butter to accompany.
5. Hard-boiled eggs with a dab of mayonnaise on salad greens.
6. Stuffed eggs. Remove yolks from hard-boiled eggs. Mix with butter and shrimp, cheese, olives, or ham, etc. Fill the whites.

7. Grated raw vegetables with French dressing (see Salads).
8. Cooked brown rice with chopped ham, peas, or mushrooms and paprika French dressing.
9. Stuffed tomatoes. Cut tops off fresh tomatoes and set aside. Remove seeds and core. Add the juice to chopped vegetables and meat or fish or cottage cheese. Fill tomatoes with mixture and put tops back on.

AVOCADO TOSSED TUNA SALAD

NO COOKING

1 medium-sized lettuce
1 small onion
1 large tomato
1 small can of tuna fish (approx. 7 oz.)
1 avocado
French Dressing (see Salads)
1 hard-boiled egg

1. Wash, dry, and break lettuce into small leaves. Place in a large salad bowl.
2. Peel the onion, then grate it finely. Cut the tomato into thin wedges.
3. Drain and flake the tuna fish.
4. Peel and pit the avocado. Cut the flesh into small pieces.
5. Add onion, tomato, avocado, and tuna to the lettuce. Toss with approximately ¼ cup French dressing.

To serve: Slice the hard-boiled egg and use as a garnish. Serves 6 people as a starter.

COTTAGE CHEESE PEARS

NO COOKING

4 firm ripe dessert pears

Dressing
¼ cup (scant) oil
2 tablespoons lemon juice
dash of salt, dry mustard
pepper

Filling
1 cup cottage cheese
½ to ¾ cup diced lean ham
3 tablespoons mayonnaise (see Salads)
1 to 3 tablespoons chopped parsley

1. Peel, core, and halve the pears.
2. Blend the oil and lemon juice with the seasonings and sprinkle over the pears to keep them from discoloring.
3. Mix the cottage cheese with the diced ham, mayonnaise, and parsley.
4. Fill the pear halves with the cottage cheese mixture.

Serve on lettuce and garnish with parsley.

PÂTÉ

COOKING TIME: 1 HOUR
OVEN TEMPERATURE: 350°F

- 1 pound calf or beef liver
- ¾ pound unsmoked (or flat) bacon pieces (fatty)
- 1 tablespoon chopped fried onions (optional)
- ¼ level teaspoon pepper
- ½ level teaspoon ground mace (optional)
- pinch of ground nutmeg
- ¼ pound thinly sliced bacon

1. Wash liver in warm water. Remove rinds from the bacon.
2. Mince liver and fatty bacon together, then pulp in an electric blender to give a smooth texture.
3. If onion is used, chop it finely and fry in a little butter or oil. Mix into meat.
4. Add pepper, mace, and nutmeg.
5. Line a straight-sided pan, mold, or cake tin with the slices of bacon and pack the liver mixture into it. Cover with foil.
6. Bake for about 1 hour. It is done when the juices from inside begin to squeeze out to the top and it shrinks away from the side of the container.

Serve with crisp whole-meal toast or green salad, or as an open sandwich on whole-meal bread or with other cold sliced meats.

SHRIMP COCKTAIL

NO COOKING

Marinade

- 6 ounces shelled and cooked shrimp
- lemon juice
- dash Tabasco
- freshly ground pepper
- shredded lettuce

Dressing

- 1 cup mayonnaise (see Salads)
- ½ small sweet red or green pepper, chopped and blanched
- 1 stick celery, chopped
- 2 teaspoons grated horseradish (optional)
- 2 tablespoons cream
- 1 teaspoon tomato purée

1. Marinate the shrimp in the juice.
2. Combine all the dressing ingredients and season to taste.
3. Place a generous tablespoon of shredded lettuce in four cocktail goblets.
4. Top with the shrimp and moisten with the dressing.

To serve: Sprinkle with paprika and decorate each serving with one or two whole shrimp and lemon wedges.

PINEAPPLE RING

NO COOKING

- 1 tablespoon gelatin
- 2 cups water
- juice of two large oranges
- 1 tablespoon wine vinegar
- 5 to 6 tablespoons diced fresh pineapple
- watercress

Cream cheese dressing

- ½ cup cream cheese
- ½ cup light cream
- salt and pepper

For the dressing, grate cheese through a strainer and beat in the cream. Season to taste. Chill.

1. Mix the gelatin with a little water. Heat gently to dissolve.
2. Mix with the rest of the water, orange juice, and vinegar. Make up to 1¼ pints (2½ cups) with water if necessary.
3. Rinse a ring mold with cold water. Pour in a little of the juices and allow to set. Arrange the pineapple on top of this and spoon over the rest of the liquid.

To serve: When set, turn out. Fill the center with watercress and serve the cream cheese dressing separately.

Variation: Use soft or puréed fruit instead of the pineapple.

Soups

A soup is a nutritious and interesting way to start a meal. All homemade soups can be eaten as long as whole-meal flour is used as the thickening agent where necessary.

Here is just a very small selection, but other kinds may easily be made using the same basic recipes.

Bran may easily be incorporated into most of the thickened soups.

BEETROOT SOUP (Borscht)

COOKING TIME: 30 MINUTES

- 4 to 6 medium-sized beetroots
- butter
- 2½ cups beef stock
- seasoning

1. Grate beetroot and fry lightly in butter in a large saucepan.
2. Add the stock and simmer gently for 30 minutes.
3. Blend the soup thoroughly and season to taste.
4. Reheat soup. Serve hot with sour cream.

Variation: This soup is also delicious if served cold with sour cream.

CONSOMMÉ (Clear Soup)

COOKING TIME: 10 MINUTES

4 ounces lean juicy beef
1 small onion
1 small carrot
5 cups brown stock
chilled shell and white of one egg
8 to 10 peppercorns
bouquet garni
blade of mace
1 clove

1. Chop the meat very fine and soak in 2 tablespoons water for 30 minutes.
2. Wash the vegetables, then chop into thick pieces.
3. Remove the fat from the stock and strain through muslin.
4. Wash and crush the eggshell and whisk the egg white slightly.
5. Place the vegetables, meat, and herbs into a muslin bag. Add to the stock with the eggshell and white.
6. Heat slowly and whisk until it boils. Boil for 5 minutes. Take off the heat and let stand for 30 minutes, tightly covered. This allows time for any solids to settle.
7. Strain through a linen cloth. Repeat if not sufficiently clear.
8. Reheat and add garnishes.

Garnishes

Finely shredded carrot and turnip cooked in salted water.
Finely diced vegetables cooked in salted water.
Cooked asparagus tips and minced mushrooms.
Tomato purée.
String beans cooked and sliced French style.

GAZPACHO

NO COOKING

2 pounds tomatoes
1 sweet green pepper
1 sweet red pepper
½ cucumber
6 small onions
1 tablespoon olive oil
1 tablespoon vinegar
1 cup cold water
1 clove of garlic, crushed
salt and pepper
1 hard-boiled egg for garnish
ice cubes

1. Purée the tomatoes.
2. Dice finely the peppers, cucumber, and onions.
3. Stir the vegetables into the tomato purée, then add the olive oil, vinegar, and cold water.
4. Add the crushed garlic and season to taste with salt and pepper. Chill well.

To serve: Place soup in individual soup bowls garnished with sieved egg yolk. Add one ice cube to each dish before serving.

FRENCH ONION SOUP

COOKING TIME: 1 HOUR 30 MINUTES

- 2 slices of fatty bacon
- 6 medium-sized onions
- 1 tablespoon whole-meal flour
- salt and pepper
- ½ teaspoon French mustard
- 4 cups beef stock
- 6 small rounds of whole-meal bread
- ½ cup grated cheese

1. Chop the bacon finely, then heat it in a deep pan until the fat runs freely.
2. Slice the onions thinly, then fry them slowly in the bacon fat.
3. Stir in the flour and seasonings and continue to cook the mixture gently.
4. Stir in the mustard and stock. Simmer until the onions are quite soft (approximately one hour's simmering is necessary to get the best results).

To serve: Toast the whole-meal bread, then sprinkle the grated cheese on the top. Grill the cheese toasts until the cheese has melted and browned. Serve each portion of soup with a cheese crouton floating on top.

TOMATO SOUP

COOKING TIME: 1 HOUR

- ¼ cup butter
- 1 large onion
- 1 large carrot
- 1 slice of bacon, finely chopped
- 2 tablespoons whole-meal flour
- 4 cups beef stock
- 1 pound ripe tomatoes
- bouquet garni
- salt and pepper

1. Melt butter in a thick-bottomed saucepan. Dice onion and carrot finely and then fry these in the butter until soft. Add the chopped bacon and cook mixture for 1 minute.
2. Mix in the whole-meal flour, and cook the mixture for 1 or 2 minutes.
3. Slowly add the meat stock, stirring all the time. Bring to boil.
4. Slice the tomatoes thinly and add to the soup.
5. Add the bouquet garni and season lightly.
6. Simmer for 50 minutes. Remove bouquet garni.
7. Blend the soup thoroughly, then taste, and add more seasonings, if necessary. Reheat and serve with whole-meal croutons.

Variation: The juice and grated rind of an orange may be added to the soup to give it a tang.

SHRIMP CHOWDER

COOKING TIME: 25 MINUTES

1 tablespoon butter
1 onion
5 potatoes
salt and pepper
1 cup boiling water
2 cups milk
1 cup shelled shrimp (fresh or frozen)

1. Melt the butter. Chop the onion finely, then fry it lightly in the butter.
2. Peel and slice the potatoes, then add them to the softened onions. Add salt, pepper, and boiling water.
3. Simmer gently for about 15 minutes, or until the potatoes are cooked.
4. Add the milk and shrimp and bring to boil.

To serve: Garnish with chopped parsley and serve with whole-meal bread rolls.

Variations: Replace shrimp with clams or corn or chopped celery.

PEA SOUP

COOKING TIME: 2 HOURS 10 MINUTES

⅔ cup split peas
1 carrot
1 turnip
1 onion
5 cups stock (ham preferably)
bouquet garni
salt and pepper
1 tablespoon whole-meal flour
1¼ cups milk

1. Soak peas overnight in water.
2. Dice vegetables. Combine peas, vegetables, stock, bouquet garni, and salt and pepper in a pan.
3. Bring to boil and simmer for 2 hours. Remove bouquet garni.
4. Season to taste. Add the flour blended with the milk. Reheat slowly.

To serve: Sprinkle with chopped parsley.

CREME VICHYSSOISE

COOKING TIME: 15 MINUTES

3 large well-blanched leeks
1 tablespoon butter
1 stick celery, sliced
3 medium-sized potatoes, sliced
3 cups jelled chicken stock
salt and pepper
¼ pint cream
chives (optional)

1. Slice the leeks thinly, discarding any green part. Lightly fry in butter until soft, without browning.
2. Add the sliced celery and potatoes and stock.
3. Season and simmer until they are soft.
4. Rub through a fine sieve or Mouli.
5. Season to taste and stir in the cream.
6. Chill.

The soup should be very smooth and bland. A few chives or snipped celery tops may be sprinkled on the top before serving.

Breads

Delicious breads and scones can be made using whole-meal flour. The recipes given use yeast or baking powder as a raising agent. Bran can be added to these quite successfully.

You will probably find whole-meal bread very different from regular bread, but once you acquire a taste for it you will not want to return to white bread.

WHOLE-MEAL BREAD

COOKING TIME: 30 TO 35 MINUTES
OVEN TEMPERATURE: 450°F

2 cups water (hand-hot)
3 level teaspoons dried yeast
1 teaspoon sugar (just to start the fermentation and make the dough rise sooner)
2 tablespoons fat
6 cups whole-meal flour
3 level teaspoons salt

To obtain water at hand temperature blend 1 part boiling water with 2 parts cold water.

1. Take 1 cup of the hand-hot water and whisk in the dried yeast and the sugar with a fork. Leave the yeast liquid to stand in a warm place for 10 to 15 minutes, or until frothy.
2. Rub the fat into the flour and add the salt.
3. Pour in the rest of the water and the yeast liquid and mix thoroughly to form a dough.
4. Take the dough and place it on a lightly floured surface. Knead the dough for 5 minutes or until it is smooth.
5. Place the dough in a lightly floured polyethylene bag and put it in a warm place for 30 minutes to let rise.
6. Take the dough, knead it lightly, then divide it into two equal pieces. Knead each piece into a smooth ball. Keep the dough in the polyethylene bag whenever it is not being handled.

7. Grease and warm two loaf pans. Shape each ball of dough to fit the pans. Place the pans into the polyethylene bag and put them in a warm place for 30 minutes or until the dough has risen ¼ to ¾ inch over the rim of the pans.
8. Remove the polyethylene bag, place the pans on the center shelf of the oven, and bake for 30 to 35 minutes. Reduce the oven temperature to 425°F after 20 minutes, if the loaves brown too quickly.
9. Cool the loaves on a wire rack.

IRISH SODA BREAD

COOKING TIME: 20 TO 30 MINUTES
OVEN TEMPERATURE: 400°F

- 2 cups whole-meal flour
- 1 level teaspoon baking soda
- ½ level teaspoon cream of tartar
- salt
- buttermilk

1. Mix dry ingredients together.
2. Add enough buttermilk to form a soft dough.
3. Roll on to a floured board.
4. Shape with hands and place in a cake tin.
5. Bake in a hot oven for 20 to 30 minutes.

Serve hot or cold, spread with butter.

Variation: Roll out to 1-inch thickness, cut into triangles, and cook for approximately 10 minutes each side on a hot griddle.

FRUIT LOAF

COOKING TIME: 50 TO 60 MINUTES
OVEN TEMPERATURE: 350°F

- ½ cup margarine
- 3 cups whole-meal flour
- 1 teaspoon mixed spice
- 4 cups mixed fruit and peel
- 1 teaspoon salt
- 1 beaten egg

Yeast mixture

- 1 cup whole-meal flour
- 1½ teaspoons dried yeast
- 1 teaspoon sugar (see Whole-meal Bread)
- 1¼ cups warm water

Yeast mixture

1. Put 1 cup flour into large mixing bowl.
2. Add yeast, sugar, and water and mix well.
3. Cover with cloth and set aside in warm place until foamy (approximately 20 minutes).

1. Blend margarine with 3 cups flour, mix in spice, fruit, and salt, add beaten egg, and finally the yeast liquid.
2. Knead dough on lightly floured board. Place in greased polyethylene bag and leave in warm place to rise until double the size.
3. Turn out dough, knock out air bubbles, and knead well.
4. Divide in two and shape into two greased 8 x 8 x 2 loaf tins. Cover each tin, leave in warm place to rise.
5. When double the size, remove cover and bake in moderate oven.

OATCAKES

COOKING TIME: 30 MINUTES
OVEN TEMPERATURE: 325°F

½ cup margarine
2 cups oatmeal
1 cup whole-meal flour
salt
3 to 4 tablespoons boiling water

1. Melt margarine.
2. Add dry ingredients and mix with water.
3. Roll out to ¼-inch thickness and cut into shapes.
4. Place on a greased baking sheet and bake for approximately 30 minutes.

Serve with butter and cheese.

DATE SCONES

COOKING TIME: 15 MINUTES
OVEN TEMPERATURE: 425°F

2 cups whole-meal flour
3 teaspoons baking powder
2 tablespoons butter
1 cup chopped dates
1 egg
milk

1. Mix flour and baking powder. Blend in butter.
2. Add chopped dates.
3. Beat egg and add to dry ingredients with enough milk to give a soft consistency.
4. Roll out to 1-inch thickness. Cut into 1½-inch rounds.
5. Place on a baking sheet and bake for approximately 15 minutes.

YOGURT WHOLE-MEAL SCONES
(Buttermilk biscuits)

COOKING TIME: 10 MINUTES
OVEN TEMPERATURE: 400°F

- 2 cups whole-meal flour
- 2 teaspoons baking powder
- ¼ teaspoon salt
- 3 tablespoons shortening
- 1¼ cups natural yogurt

1. Mix the whole-meal flour, baking powder, and salt together.
2. Blend the shortening with the flour until the mixture resembles fine bread crumbs.
3. Stir in the yogurt and form the mixture into a soft dough.
4. Roll out the dough on a floured board until it is 1 inch thick. Cut into 1½-inch rounds and place on a greased baking sheet.
5. Bake at 400°F for 10 minutes.

Serve with butter and cheese; or whipped cream and mashed bananas.

CHEESE SCONES

COOKING TIME: 10 MINUTES
OVEN TEMPERATURE: 425°F

- 2 cups whole-meal flour
- 2 teaspoons baking powder
- ¼ cup butter
- 1½ cups grated cheese
- salt and pepper
- ½ teaspoon dry mustard
- ½ cup milk
- a little cayenne pepper

1. Grease and flour a baking sheet.
2. Sieve flour and baking powder. Blend in the butter until the mixture resembles fine bread crumbs.
3. Add 1 cup grated cheese, the seasonings (except the cayenne pepper), and mix well.
4. Mix to a fairly stiff dough with milk.
5. Turn on to a floured board and knead lightly.
6. Roll out to 1-inch thickness. Cut into 1½-inch rounds and place on the baking sheet.
7. Sprinkle the remaining ½ cup cheese on top and cayenne pepper sparingly.
8. Bake in the hottest part of the oven until the cheese topping is crisp and the scones well risen.

Serve hot or cold with butter.

Pastry

When you make any type of pastry with whole-meal flour, you will need slightly more water than with white flour. On the other hand, the texture tends to be harder so make sure you don't add too much liquid.

We have suggested a few very basic pastry recipes, but why not try your favorite ones substituting the whole-meal flour for white?

AMERICAN PIE PASTRY

- ½ cup (generous) lard or other shortening
- 2 tablespoons cold water
- salt
- 2 cups whole-meal flour
- 2 teaspoons baking powder

1. Cream the fat and water with a pinch of salt.
2. Mix the flour and baking powder, sprinkle over the mixture and mix to a rough paste.
3. Chill for 30 minutes.
4. Turn onto a floured board, knead lightly, and use for fruit pies.

SHORTCRUST PASTRY

- 2 cups whole-meal flour
- salt
- ½ cup butter or other shortening
- 3 to 4 tablespoons water

1. Mix the flour with a pinch of salt in a bowl.
2. Rub the fat into the flour until the mixture resembles fine bread crumbs.
3. Add the water and mix with a knife. Add a little more cold water if necessary.
4. The dough should be firm but not sticky.
5. Turn out onto a floured board and knead lightly. Chill before using.

Variations: Omit ½ cup flour and add 1 cup grated cheese. Add 1 egg yolk in exchange for some of the water. Use this paste for cheese straws, etc.

FLAKY PASTRY

2 cups whole-meal flour
salt
2 teaspoons baking powder
⅓ cup shortening
⅓ cup butter
a few drops lemon juice
water to mix

1. Mix the flour, salt, and baking powder in a bowl.
2. Blend the shortening and butter together and divide into three equal portions. Chill.
3. Blend a third of the fat into the flour.
4. Add the lemon juice and some water, mix with a knife to form a dry but firm dough.
5. Turn onto a lightly floured board, knead until smooth and roll into an oblong.
6. Dot the uppermost two-thirds of the pastry with the remaining fat (cut into small pieces). Fold pastry over to form three layers, i.e., pastry/fat/pastry/fat/pastry. Seal the edges.
7. Half turn the pastry to bring the sealed ends in front of you. Roll again to an oblong and repeat the folding and rolling procedure twice more.
8. Chill for 10 to 15 minutes. Roll out and fold once more.
9. Chill once again before using.

Variation: Use with sweet or other fillings.

CHOUX PASTRY

½ cup water
¼ cup butter
1 generous cup of whole-meal flour
2 eggs
vanilla extract

1. Bring the water and butter to the boil. Remove from heat.
2. Add the flour and return to the stove to cook, beating until smooth for 1 to 2 minutes.
3. Allow to cool slightly.
4. Lightly beat or whisk the eggs and gradually beat into the flour mixture, a little at a time. Add flavoring if required.
5. The mixture should be smooth and have a shiny appearance.

Suggestions

Spoon dough on to greased baking sheet and bake at 375°F for 20 minutes until firm. Fill with fresh or stewed fruit. Serve with cream or fruit purée sauce.

Add fillings such as thick shrimp or mushroom sauce, etc.

Sauces and Stuffings

A well-made sauce improves both the flavor and appearance of a dish. It is very simple and quick to prepare and may be served with a wide variety of foods. Some suggestions are made in this section.

The stuffing recipes given are particularly good accompaniments to poultry, but will enhance any other plain meat dish.

Bran mixes extremely well into both sauces and stuffings.

BASIC WHITE SAUCE

COOKING TIME: 10 MINUTES

- ¼ cup butter or margarine
- ½ cup whole-meal flour
- 2½ cups milk or milk and stock
- seasoning (omit for sweet sauces)

1. Melt butter, stir in flour until fat is absorbed.
2. Add milk gradually, stirring briskly until boiling and the mixture thickens.
3. Boil slowly for 3 to 5 minutes, continuing to stir.
4. Add seasoning to taste.

SAVORY (NON-SWEET) SAUCES

Use Basic White Sauce with seasoning.

Variations

Anchovy Sauce:
 1 tablespoon anchovy paste and fish stock.

Caper Sauce:
 1 tablespoon capers

Cheese Sauce:
 2 tablespoons grated cheese

Dutch Sauce:
 1 raw egg yolk, a few drops of vinegar, 1 teaspoon lemon juice

Egg Sauce:
 1 chopped hard-boiled egg

Mustard Sauce:
 1 tablespoon dry mustard and 2 tablespoons vinegar

Onion Sauce:
 2 large cooked onions, chopped

Parsley Sauce:
 1 tablespoon freshly chopped parsley

Shrimp Sauce:
 2 tablespoons shrimp, chopped

Serve with fish, meat, or with other recipes as suggested.

CURRY SAUCE

COOKING TIME: 45 MINUTES

- 2 medium-sized onions
- 1 tablespoon butter or other shortening
- 2 teaspoons curry powder
- ½ teaspoon curry paste
- 2 teaspoons whole-meal flour
- 1 clove of garlic
- 1 cup stock or coconut milk
- salt
- a little cayenne pepper
- 1 tablespoon relish (see Salads)
- 1 tablespoon cream

1. Finely chop onions and fry in melted butter until golden brown.
2. Add curry powder, paste, and flour. Cook for 5 minutes.
3. Add garlic, pour in stock or coconut milk and bring to the boil.
4. Add seasonings, relish, and simmer for 30 to 40 minutes.
5. If desired, add cream immediately before use.

Serve with hard-boiled eggs, or combine with diced chicken and serve cold with rice salad.

CREOLE SAUCE

COOKING TIME: 30 MINUTES

- 1 tablespoon butter
- 1 small chopped onion
- ½ medium sweet green pepper, diced
- 1 medium can of tomatoes
- ¼ teaspoon Tabasco
- ½ teaspoon salt

1. Melt butter in a saucepan. Add onion and pepper; fry until tender but not browned.
2. Add tomatoes, Tabasco, and salt. Bring to boil, then simmer for approximately 20 minutes.

Serve with steak, pork, or pasta.

HORSERADISH SAUCE

NO COOKING

- 1 tablespoon vinegar
- ½ teaspoon mustard
- salt and pepper
- 2 tablespoons (heaping) fresh-grated horseradish
- generous cup of heavy cream

1. Mix vinegar, seasonings, and horseradish together.
2. Whip the cream lightly and mix carefully with the other ingredients.
3. Adjust the seasoning to taste.

Serve with roast beef.

BARBECUE SAUCE

COOKING TIME: 10 MINUTES

1 small onion
1 stalk celery
2 teaspoons (level) dry mustard
1 teaspoon (level) salt
½ teaspoon (level) pepper
2 teaspoons tomato paste
2 tablespoons lemon juice
3 teaspoons Worcestershire or soy sauce
½ cup water
2 teaspoons vinegar

1. Peel and chop the onion. Wash and chop the celery finely.
2. Mix mustard, salt, and pepper with the tomato paste and the liquids.
3. Fry onions in butter or oil. Add celery and other ingredients. Simmer for 10 minutes.

Serve hot or cold.

TOMATO SAUCE

COOKING TIME: 45 MINUTES

2 tablespoons butter
2 tablespoons whole-meal flour
1 cup beef stock
1½ cups tomatoes (fresh or canned)
bouquet garni
salt and pepper

1. Melt 1 tablespoon butter in a saucepan. Add the flour, mix, and pour into the stock. Bring to boil.
2. Roughly chop the tomatoes.
3. Add them with the bouquet garni and seasonings and any tomato juice left over.
4. Cover and simmer for ½ hour.
5. Strain, pressing well to extract the juice.
6. Season to taste and reheat.
7. Beat in the second tablespoon of butter before serving.

BREAD SAUCE

COOKING TIME: 30 MINUTES

1 medium-sized onion
2 cloves
1½ cups milk
salt
1 cup whole-meal bread crumbs
1 tablespoon butter

1. Peel the onion and stick cloves into it; place in a saucepan of milk and salt. Bring to the boil and leave to stand for 20 minutes.
2. Add the bread crumbs and the butter, mixing well.
3. Cook slowly for 15 minutes, then remove the onion.

Serve hot with turkey or chicken.

MINT SAUCE

NO COOKING

2 tablespoons chopped mint
1½ tablespoons vinegar

1. Finely chop the mint, after removing the stalks.
2. Add vinegar, allow to stand for ½ hour.

Serve with lamb.

TARTARE SAUCE

NO COOKING

1¼ cups mayonnaise (see Salad recipes)
1 tablespoon chopped gherkins
3 teaspoons chopped capers
1 tablespoon finely chopped tarragon and chervil

1. Finely chop all ingredients and add them to the mayonnaise.
2. Mix well. Thin to the required consistency with a little vinegar (if necessary).
3. Allow to stand for a short time before use, to allow the flavors to blend.

Serve with any fish.

SWEET SAUCES

ORANGE SAUCE

COOKING TIME: 10 MINUTES

Basic White Sauce
1 egg yolk
grated rind of 1 orange
juice of 2 oranges

1. Make basic white sauce as in recipe.
2. Add egg yolk carefully and cook gently for 1 minute.
3. Add rind and juice of orange.

Serve with roast duck or use as a sauce with suitable puddings.

CUSTARD SAUCE

COOKING TIME: APPROX. 10 MINUTES

1¼ cups milk
1 teaspoon vanilla extract or a strip of lemon rind
1 egg

1. Heat the milk and lemon rind (or vanilla extract) but do not boil.
2. Pour on to well-beaten egg, stirring continuously.
3. Return to pan and cook over hot water until the sauce coats the back of the spoon thinly.
4. Strain and cool, stirring occasionally, or serve hot if desired.

Serve with suitable puddings.

APPLE SAUCE

COOKING TIME: 30 MINUTES

- 1 pound apples, pared, cored, and cut up
- 1 tablespoon butter or margarine
- lemon juice to flavor (optional)

1. Cook apples gently to a pulp, using as little water as possible.
2. Beat with a wooden spoon or blend to make a purée.
3. Add the butter mixing well, then the lemon juice, if used.

Serve with pork.

FRUIT SAUCE

Any suitable fruit, e.g., strawberries, raspberries, plums, or gooseberries, can be blended with a little water and served as a hot or cold sauce.

STUFFINGS

CHESTNUT STUFFING

- 1 pound chestnuts
- 1 cup ham stock or milk
- ½ cup ham or bacon, chopped
- 1½ cups fresh whole-meal bread crumbs
- 1 teaspoon chopped parsley
- 1 tablespoon butter
- grated lemon rind
- salt and pepper
- 1 egg

1. Make a slit in both ends of the chestnuts and boil in water for about 10 minutes. Taking a few at a time from the water, skin them.
2. Put the shelled nuts into a pan with enough stock or milk just to cover and simmer gently until tender. Mash the chestnuts or press them through a sieve.
3. Mash the finely chopped ham or bacon into the chestnut mixture, add bread crumbs, finely chopped parsley, melted butter, and grated lemon rind.
4. Season with salt and pepper, bind with beaten egg.

Use as stuffing for turkey, chicken, or other poultry.

SAGE AND ONION STUFFING

2 large onions
2 teaspoons dried sage or 4 to 5 fresh sage leaves
1 tablespoon butter
2 cups fresh whole-meal bread crumbs

1. Peel onions, boil in water for 5 minutes.
2. Drain off water, add fresh boiling water, and cook until tender.
3. Drain well, cool, chop onion finely, add to all other ingredients and mix well.

Use as poultry stuffing.

WALNUT STUFFING

1 pound cooked potatoes
¼ cup melted butter
1 beaten egg
1 cup finely chopped walnuts

1. Rice the potatoes.
2. Add the melted butter, egg, and nuts. Mix well.

Use as stuffing for duck.

Fish

Most fish dishes need little modification. Remember always to use the whole-meal substitutes for regular flour and bread when making sauces and batter and when using bread crumbs. Apart from this, continue with all your favorite recipes and experiment with the following suggestions.

TUNA RISOTTO

COOKING TIME: 45 MINUTES

1 small onion
1 large can tuna
1½ cups long grain brown rice
celery, green pepper, sweet corn, etc.
4 fresh tomatoes, or 1 small can of tomatoes
tomato purée
seasoning

1. Chop onion and fry gently in juice drained from can of tuna.
2. Add rice and fry for a few minutes, stirring all the time.

3. Chop vegetables and tomatoes fairly small and add to frying mixture.
4. Gradually pour in 2½ cups hot water. Cover pan and simmer for 35 to 40 minutes until the rice has swollen and absorbed the liquid. Stir frequently, adding a little more liquid if the mixture gets too dry.
5. Flake tuna and add to the mixture with the tomato purée. Season to taste and cook for a further 5 minutes.

Serve hot with a green salad. Especially good if tossed in French Dressing immediately before serving.

TUNA CRUMBLE

COOKING TIME: 25 TO 30 MINUTES
OVEN TEMPERATURE: 400°F

Filling

- 1 can tuna fish
- 1 hard-boiled egg
- 2 large tomatoes
- ½ cup mushrooms
- ½ cup milk

Topping

- ¾ cup whole-meal flour
- ¼ cup margarine
- ½ to ¾ cup grated cheese
- salt and pepper
- paprika

1. Grease a pie dish and layer tuna, sliced egg, and sliced tomato into it.
2. Slice mushrooms on top and pour milk over. Season.
3. Make topping by blending the margarine into the flour. Add grated cheese and seasoning and sprinkle over mixture in pie dish.
4. Sprinkle with paprika and bake in hot oven.

Variations

Ground meat and onion.
Chopped chicken, corn, and celery.
Baked fish in milk, with onion and mushrooms.

FISH STEAKS WITH MUSHROOMS

COOKING TIME: 30 MINUTES
OVEN TEMPERATURE: 350-400°F

- 4 cod- or swordfish steaks
- seasoning
- 1 onion
- 1 cup (heaping) mushrooms

1. Season fish with salt and pepper.
2. Chop onion and mushrooms finely and sprinkle over steaks.
3. Wrap each steak in well-greased paper or foil and place in a flat ovenproof dish.
4. Bake in oven, and when cooked, remove the paper.
5. Pour off the liquid and make into a sauce (see Basic White Sauce recipe), adding chopped parsley, if desired.
6. Pour sauce over the steaks to serve.

COD WITH ORANGE AND WALNUTS

COOKING TIME: 20-30 MINUTES
OVEN TEMPERATURE: 350°F

- 2 tablespoons butter or oil
- 1½ cups fresh whole-meal bread crumbs
- 1 finely chopped clove of garlic (optional)
- ¼ cup finely chopped walnuts
- grated peel and juice of 1 medium orange
- 4 cod- or swordfish steaks (4 to 6 ounces each)
- salt and pepper

1. Heat butter or oil in pan, stir in bread crumbs, garlic if used, walnuts, and orange peel.
2. Let stand over low heat, stirring frequently until fat has been absorbed by crumbs.
3. Sprinkle fish with salt and pepper, stand in greased shallow heatproof dish.
4. Moisten with orange juice. Cover with bread crumb mixture.
5. Bake uncovered in center of moderate oven for 20 to 30 minutes.

Serve with any vegetable or salad.

CREOLE FISH SPECIAL

COOKING TIME: 30 MINUTES
OVEN TEMPERATURE: 350°F

- 1 tablespoon butter
- 2 pounds fillet of fresh haddock or cod
- 1 cup sour cream
- 3 tablespoons milk
- ¼ teaspoon Tabasco
- ½ teaspoon (level) salt
- 1 tablespoon (level) paprika
- ¼ cup (1 ounce) finely grated Cheddar cheese
- 4 tablespoons (level) fresh whole-meal bread crumbs
- lemon slices

1. Grease an ovenproof dish with a little of the butter, and place fish in it.
2. Mix together sour cream, milk, Tabasco, salt, paprika, and cheese. Spread over fish, sprinkle bread crumbs on top, and dot with remaining butter.
3. Bake uncovered in a moderate oven until fish is tender.
4. Garnish with lemon.

Serve with any hot vegetables and baked potatoes.

Meats

Meat dishes do not pose much of a problem as all types of meat, served hot or cold, are suitable. All gravies and sauces can be thickened with whole-meal flour and you can use whole-meal pastry for pies, toppings, dumplings, etc.

Bran can easily be incorporated into any of these items.

HAMBURGERS

COOKING TIME: 15 MINUTES

8 ounces ground beef
1 large potato, grated
1 cup finely chopped onion
dash of Tabasco
1 tablespoon chopped parsley
pinch of mixed herbs
seasoning
1 egg, beaten
browned whole-meal bread crumbs

1. Mix the beef with the potatoes and onion. Add flavorings and seasonings and mix well.
2. Fork in beaten egg until mixture binds together.
3. Form into 4 firm rounds and coat with bread crumbs.
4. Grill slowly until cooked.

Serve with fried sliced onions in warm whole-meal buns.

Suggestions: Serve with grilled apple rings or with slice of cheese grilled until brown, or with barbecue sauce or tomato sauce.

BARBECUED SPARERIBS

COOKING TIME: 1½ HOURS
OVEN TEMPERATURE: 400°F

4 portions thick spareribs (4 ribs a person)
Barbecue Sauce

1. Place chops in wide shallow casserole and bake uncovered for about 30 minutes until well browned. Pour off excess fat.
2. Meanwhile prepare the Barbecue Sauce (see recipe), but do not cook it. Pour it over the chops. Cover and bake for about ¾ hour.

Serve with baked potatoes and green vegetables.

ROAST BEEF (of Olde Englande)

This is the traditional English Sunday lunch. Choose a suitably sized joint of beef (allowing 8 to 12 ounces raw meat (including bone) each) and roast in the usual way.

Serve with the following accompaniments:

Roast Potatoes

1. Scrub the potatoes.
2. Roll them in the hot fat in the roasting pan round the joint or heat ¼ cup fat in a separate pan.
3. Cook for approximately 45 minutes at 375°F.
4. If you like roast potatoes "floury," parboil them in salted water for 10 minutes first.

Gravy

1. When the meat is cooked, pour away all the fat except for about 1 tablespoon.
2. For a fairly thin gravy gradually blend in 1 tablespoon whole-meal flour.
3. Gradually work in about 1 cup of water or stock, bring to the boil and cook until thickened.
4. Strain and use.

Yorkshire Pudding

COOKING TIME: 20 MINUTES
OVEN TEMPERATURE: 450°-475°F

1 cup whole-meal flour
salt
1 egg
1⅓ cups milk

1. Combine flour and salt and add the egg.
2. Gradually work in the milk to form a "batter" consistency.
3. When you remove the roast beef from the oven, turn the heat up to 475°F.
4. Preheat a shallow or Yorkshire pudding pan with a tablespoon of fat in it.
5. Pour batter into the pan and place on top of shelf of hot oven.
6. Traditionally Yorkshire pudding is served with gravy as a separate course, but nowadays it is usually served as an accompaniment to roast beef.

HORSERADISH SAUCE. See recipe in Sauce section.

Roast beef should be served with at least two vegetables: one green vegetable, e.g., cabbage, sprouts, cauliflower, and one root vegetable, e.g., rutabaga, carrot, parsnips. Parsnips may be roasted along with the potatoes, but should be parboiled for 5 to 10 minutes first, unless they are very young and tender.

DEEP BAYOU MEAT LOAF

COOKING TIME: 1¼ HOURS
OVEN TEMPERATURE: 350°F

- 1 cup tomato juice
- 1 teaspoon Tabasco
- 1 egg, beaten
- 1½ cups fresh whole-meal bread crumbs
- 1 cup onion, finely chopped
- 2 tablespoons (level) parsley
- ¼ teaspoon (level) thyme
- 1½ teaspoons (level) salt
- 2 pounds ground beef

1. Mix all ingredients together well.
2. Turn into a greased loaf tin (approx. 9 x 5 x 3 inches).
3. Bake for 1¼ hours in a moderate oven (350°F).
4. Serve hot or cold with salad.

CORNISH PASTY

COOKING TIME: 1 HOUR
OVEN TEMPERATURE: 400°F

- 1 recipe whole-meal Flaky Pastry
- 1 pound braising beef
- 1 large onion
- 1 rutabaga (if available)
- 2 large potatoes
- salt and pepper
- 4 tablespoons gravy or water
- whole-meal flour
- 1 egg, beaten or milk

1. Make pastry (see Flaky Pastry recipe). Cut into 4.
2. Roll out one piece to size of a dinner plate.
3. Cut meat into very small pieces. Chop the onion, grate rutabaga, and dice potatoes.
4. Spread ingredients over center of pastry, starting with a layer of meat, then onion, rutabaga, potato, meat, and so on. Pour over gravy or water.
5. Season and sprinkle with whole-meal flour.
6. Close and squeeze edges; make tucks in pastry to keep the edges together.
7. Brush with beaten egg or milk. Place on a flat baking sheet.
8. Bake in a hot oven for 1 hour.

Serve hot or cold. No other vegetables are necessary.

LIVER AND BACON CASSEROLE

COOKING TIME: 1½ HOURS
OVEN TEMPERATURE: 300°F

¾ pound liver
4 ounces bacon
4 ounces mushrooms
salt and pepper
1 cup water

Topping
1 ounce margarine
1 cup whole-meal bread crumbs
chopped parsley
salt and pepper

1. Grease an ovenproof dish.
2. Place layers of sliced liver, chopped bacon, and sliced mushrooms in it.
3. Season, and add 1 cup water.
4. Prepare topping by rubbing fat into crumbs and adding parsley and seasoning.
5. Sprinkle over other ingredients.
6. Cover and bake.
7. Remove lid after 1 hour to allow top to become brown and crisp.

N.B. Extra bran may be added to the topping, if desired.

LAMB KEBABS

COOKING TIME: 16 MINUTES

1 pound fillet of lamb
½ cup natural yogurt
1 tablespoon lemon juice
1 tablespoon (level) finely grated onion
½ teaspoon (level) salt
4 small onions or shallots
8 slices of bacon
8 small tomatoes
8 button mushrooms
butter or oil
1 cup Brown Rice, boiled (see recipe)

1. Cut lamb into 1-inch cubes. Combine yogurt, lemon juice, grated onion, and salt together. Toss lamb cubes into this mixture until well coated. Cover and chill for at least 3 hours, turning frequently.
2. Cook whole onions in boiling salted water for 10 minutes, drain, and halve.
3. Cut bacon slices in half. Roll up each one.
4. Put lamb onto 4 skewers alternately with halved onions, bacon rolls, tomatoes, and mushrooms.
5. Brush well with melted butter or oil. Broil in preheated oven for 8 minutes.
6. Brush with more fat. Broil 8 minutes more.
7. Serve with Brown Rice.

CHICKEN MAJORCA

COOKING TIME: 45 MINUTES

- 1 roasting chicken (2½ pounds dressed weight)
- 1 tablespoon oil
- ⅛ cup (1 ounce) butter
- 1 onion (large)
- 1 tablespoon (level) whole-meal flour
- 2 cups chicken stock
- salt and pepper
- bouquet garni
- 1 red sweet pepper
- 1 large orange
- 10 to 12 small green olives
- chopped parsley

1. Cut the chicken into parts. Heat the oil and butter in a frying pan to steaming point and place the pieces in it. Sauté until a good golden brown. Take out the pieces.
2. Thinly slice the onion and sauté until slightly browned.
3. Stir in the flour and stock. Bring to boil.
4. Season the gravy, add the bouquet garni, and simmer for 20 to 30 minutes, tightly covered. Then take out the bouquet garni.
5. Meanwhile lightly fry the pepper, place in cold water, and remove the skin. Cut into thin slices, removing the seeds.
6. Cut all the rind and pith from the orange, and slice. Pit the olives.

To Serve: Arrange pieces of chicken on a serving dish. Garnish with parsley. Add the pepper, olives, and orange to the gravy. Bring to a boil and cook well for a few minutes, then spoon over the dish.

Serve with banana or corn fritters.

CRUNCHY CHICKEN

COOKING TIME: 15 MINUTES
OVEN TEMPERATURE: 350°F

- ½ cup butter
- ¾ pound cooked, diced chicken
- 8 ounces cooked broccoli spears
- 2 tablespoons whole-meal flour
- 1¼ cups chicken stock
- 1 small can evaporated milk
- ½ cup grated cheese
- seasoning
- ½ cup whole-meal bread crumbs
- ½ cup chopped nuts

1. Grease a shallow ovenproof dish with half the butter.
2. Cover the bottom with the chicken, and top with the broccoli.
3. Melt the remaining butter in a pan. Stir in the flour and cook for 1 minute.
4. Slowly add the chicken stock, beating well to avoid any lumps. Allow to thicken.
5. Take off the heat. Add the evaporated milk and half the grated cheese.
6. Put back on to heat until cheese is melted. Season. Pour the sauce over the broccoli and chicken.
7. Mix the remaining cheese, bread crumbs, and nuts together, and sprinkle on top.
8. Bake in a moderate oven until bubbly and brown.

Eggs and Cheese

Eggs and cheese can be used in many ways either on their own or to add interest to other dishes.

As a snack or in place of a dessert, have fresh fruit and a variety of cheeses. Try hard-boiled eggs with Cheese or Curry Sauce (see Sauce recipes) or make Welsh or Buck Rarebit with whole-meal bread as a base. Many egg and cheese recipes include pastry or a thickened sauce. Use whole-meal flour in place of regular flour or corn flour and they will be just as successful.

A variety of more ambitious dishes has been included in this section.

PIZZA

COOKING TIME: 20 MINUTES
OVEN TEMPERATURE: 400°F

Dough

- 2 cups whole-meal flour
- 1 teaspoon (level) salt
- ¼ pint milk and water mixed
- 1 teaspoon dried yeast
- 1 teaspoon sugar (see Whole-meal Bread)
- 1 large egg
- 2 ounces softened butter

Filling

- 1 tablespoon cooking oil
- 2 medium onions
- 1 14-ounce-can tomatoes
- 1 teaspoon dried marjoram
- salt and pepper
- 4 ounces Cheddar cheese, sliced
- 1 small can anchovy fillets
- 16 black olives

To Make the Dough

1. Mix flour and salt and leave in a bowl in a warm place.
2. Warm milk and water over low heat. Add to yeast and sugar and whisk with a fork. Let stand 10 to 15 minutes to dissolve.
3. Make a hollow in the center of the flour. Beat the egg and add it and the yeast mixture to the flour.
4. Using your hands gradually mix in flour from the sides to form a soft dough.
5. Turn onto a floured board and knead for 5 minutes.
6. Spread the dough out a little and place the butter in the center. Knead the dough again until all the butter has been thoroughly incorporated.
7. Put the dough in a greased bowl, cover with wax paper, and leave in a warm place for about 40 minutes, until it has doubled in bulk.

To Make the Filling

1. Heat the oil in a frying pan. Peel and slice the onions and fry until just turning brown.
2. Add the tomatoes and marjoram. Increase the heat and bring the mixture to a boil. Boil rapidly for 20 minutes, to a fairly thick consistency, stirring occasionally.
3. Season to taste.
4. When dough is ready, knead again lightly and divide into 4 pieces.
5. Knead each piece into a round shape, place on greased baking sheet, and press out to 4½-5-inch rounds.
6. Divide the filling evenly among the dough, and spread to within ½ inch of the edges.
7. Cover the filling with thin slices of cheese.
8. Cut each anchovy fillet in half lengthwise and lay them crisscross on top. Pit and halve the olives and arrange 8 pieces around each pizza.
9. Let stand in a warm place for 15 minutes to rise.
10. Bake in hot oven.

Serve hot.

QUICK BREAD PIZZA

COOKING TIME: 5 TO 10 MINUTES

- 4 slices whole-meal bread
- 2 ounces tomato purée
- 3 to 4 ounces boiled bacon, grilled bacon pieces, *or* leftover cooked meat
- 2 tomatoes
- 4 ounces grated cheese
- 2 teaspoons Italian seasoning (mix together: dried oregano, thyme, basil, sage, and pepper)

1. Toast bread on one side.
2. Spread with tomato purée on untoasted side.
3. Place 1 slice of boiled bacon on each piece of bread.
4. Slice tomatoes, arrange on top of meat, and cover with grated cheese. Sprinkle with herbs.
5. Grill until cheese bubbles.

Serve hot with green salad.

GNOCCHI PARISIENNE

COOKING TIME: 20 MINUTES
OVEN TEMPERATURE: 375°F

- 1 cup milk
- ½ cup butter
- 1½ cups whole-meal flour
- 4 eggs
- 1 cup grated cheese
- salt and pepper

1. Boil the milk and butter together. Add the flour and beat with a wooden spoon until smooth. Allow to cool.
2. Beat in the eggs one at a time. Add half the cheese.
3. Season.
4. Put small tablespoonfuls of the mixture into simmering, salted water for approximately 12 minutes.
5. Drain and arrange in one layer on a buttered ovenproof dish.
6. Sprinkle with the rest of the cheese and bake until crisp and golden.

QUICHE LORRAINE

COOKING TIME: 30 MINUTES
OVEN TEMPERATURE: 350°F

Pastry
- 1½ cups (6 ounces) whole-meal flour
- salt
- ½ cup (4 ounces) butter
- cold water to mix

Filling
- 1 egg and 1 yolk
- ¼ cup (1 ounce) grated cheese
- ½ cup (generous) cream or milk
- seasoning
- ½ ounce butter
- 2 ounces bacon, diced
- ½ cup chopped onion

1. Prepare pastry and line a 7-inch flan ring.
2. Prepare filling by beating eggs in a bowl, adding the cheese, cream or milk, and seasoning.
3. Melt butter in a pan and add the diced bacon and onion. Cook slowly until golden.
4. Add this to egg mixture.
5. Mix and pour into the pastry shell.
6. Bake until firm (approximately 30 minutes) in a moderate oven.

Suggestions

Omit the bacon and add asparagus tips.

Add sliced tomato and sliced green sweet peppers.

Top with sliced zucchini. Cover with more grated cheese and bake.

Add corn to the mixture.

Try serving with a tomato sauce.

Make this dish into a dessert by omitting bacon and cheese, onion, and seasoning and adding fresh apples or soft fruit as the filling for the pastry.

EGGS MOLLET FLORENTINE

COOKING TIME: 15 MINUTES

- 2 pounds spinach
- 1 ounce butter
- 5 to 6 eggs
- grated cheese

Mornay Sauce

- 1 tablespoon butter
- ¼ cup whole-meal flour
- 1 cup milk
- ¼ cup grated cheese
- ¼ cup Parmesan cheese

1. Cook the spinach in boiling, salted water. Drain, dry on paper towel. Return to heat, and toss with butter. Keep warm.
2. Prepare the Mornay Sauce (see Basic White Sauce).
3. Poach the eggs in a little water.
4. Arrange spinach on a serving dish.
5. Place the eggs on top.
6. Cover with Mornay Sauce.
7. Sprinkle with extra grated cheese.
8. Brown under broiler.

Vegetables

Vegetables are an important part of the diet, and good helpings should be included daily. Have them cooked or raw, and where possible, eat skins, seeds, or stalks.

The recipes will give you some examples of how to use vegetables more imaginatively.

RATATOUILLE

(For 6 servings)

COOKING TIME: 1 HOUR
OVEN TEMPERATURE: 325°F

- 1 large eggplant
- 2 onions
- 1 sweet green pepper
- 1 sweet red pepper
- ½ pound tomatoes (fresh or canned)
- 4 small zucchini
- cooking oil
- garlic salt

1. Prepare the vegetables and cut them into neat slices.
2. Heat some cooking oil in a pan, then fry the vegetables gently to soften them.
3. Transfer the vegetables to an ovenproof dish, season them with garlic salt, cover tightly, and then cook for approximately 1 hour at 325°F.

Serve with roast beef or veal and other main course dishes.

SUMMER SQUASH

COOKING TIME: 15 TO 20 MINUTES
OVEN TEMPERATURE: 400°F

young summer squash
grated cheese
salt and pepper
butter

1. Slice young summer squash with skin and seeds as well into greased pie dish.
2. Sprinkle grated cheese on slices and top.
3. Add salt and pepper and dot with butter.
4. Place in hot oven for 15 to 20 minutes, until cheese is melted and brown.

Serve as main dish with tossed salad or as a vegetable.

STUFFED SWEET GREEN PEPPERS

COOKING TIME: 1½ TO 2 HOURS
OVEN TEMPERATURE: 350°F

5 large sweet green peppers
1 cup onion, diced
1 clove garlic
salt
½ cup mushrooms
½ cup long-grain Brown Rice
½ cup butter
2 cups ham stock
seasoning
4 ounces cooked ham
1 to 2 cups Tomato Sauce (see recipe)

1. Cut the tops off the peppers, scoop out the seeds, and core.
2. Parboil and cool.
3. Chop the onion finely, crush the garlic with the salt, and slice the mushrooms.
4. Sauté the onion in two-thirds of the butter until soft. Add the garlic and mushrooms and after 2 minutes the rice.
5. Fry for a minute, add the stock, and bring to the boil.
6. Season, cover and put into a moderate oven until the rice is cooked (40 to 50 minutes) and the stock absorbed.
7. Shred the ham and mix into the rice with the rest of the butter.
8. Fill the peppers with this mixture, arrange in a well-buttered deep baking dish, and spoon over the tomato sauce.
9. Cover with a lid and cook in a moderate oven for 40 to 50 minutes.
10. Serve in the baking dish.

CORN FRITTERS

COOKING TIME: 25 MINUTES

- 5 tablespoons corn kernels
- 1 cup fresh whole-meal bread crumbs
- 2 eggs
- 1 tablespoon thick cream
- salt and pepper
- ½ teaspoon baking powder
- oil or butter for frying

1. Cook the kernels until just tender, drain, and heat with a little butter. Put into a bowl.
2. When cool, stir in the crumbs. Separate the yolks and whites, blend the yolks with the cream and add to the corn.
3. Season well, and add the baking powder.
4. Whip the whites stiffly and fold into the mixture.
5. Heat the oil and fry the mixture in small tablespoons, turning when brown on one side.
6. Drain and serve with Tomato Sauce or as an accompaniment to chicken or veal.

BOSTON BAKED BEANS

COOKING TIME: 5 HOURS
OVEN TEMPERATURE: 250°F

- 1 pound dried haricot beans, pea beans, yellow-eyed, or your preferred beans for this purpose
- water to cover
- 2 large tomatoes
- 1 to 2 teaspoons mustard
- seasoning
- 12 ounces fat salt pork
- 1 to 2 onions

1. Soak the beans overnight in cold water.
2. Simmer 10 to 15 minutes.
3. Strain and save 1½ cups of the liquid.
4. Simmer this with tomatoes to make a thin sauce.
5. Add mustard and seasoning.
6. Dice pork and slice onions thinly.
7. Put beans, pork, and onions in deep casserole.
8. Pour tomato sauce over and mix well. Allow plenty of space for beans to swell.
9. Cover tightly and cook in slow oven. You may need to add a little extra water if the beans become dry after 2 or 3 hours.

This dish may be served on its own or as an accompaniment.

Variations

Omit the pork and add 1 or 2 crushed cloves of garlic.

Why not try a different sort of dried bean in place of haricot, e.g., black eye, butter, red kidney, or lentils?

Pancakes

The basic pancake batter is very easy to make using whole-meal flour.

However, some skill is needed to produce an alternative to maple syrup as an accompaniment for the pancakes.

Fresh and stewed fruit provide the best substitute, and of course, bacon, eggs, ham, etc. may also be served.

Some suggestions are made for more interesting varieties of pancakes.

PANCAKE BATTER

1 cup whole-meal flour
salt
1 egg
1¼ cups milk

1. Sift flour and salt into a bowl. Make a well in the center and break the egg into it. Gradually beat in the milk until smooth.
2. Let the batter stand for ½ hour before making the pancakes.
3. Grease an omelet pan well and heat thoroughly. Pour a little batter into the hot pan spreading it to cover the bottom of the pan.
4. Flip, when brown, to cook the other side. Remove from the pan and stack. (Makes 8 pancakes.)

Bran may be added to the batter before cooking.

Serve with various fillings as suggested below. Fill and roll up. Place in a serving dish and put in oven to warm through.

SAVORY PANCAKES

Pancake batter (as above)

Fillings

Chicken and Rice:

4 ounces cooked chicken or turkey (diced)
1 cup cooked brown long-grain rice
2 tablespoons chopped sweet green peppers
Basic White Sauce (see Sauce recipes)

Combine all ingredients and fill pancakes.

Ham, Corn, and Peas:

1 cup cooked diced ham
1 cup cooked corn
½ cup cooked peas
Basic White Sauce (see Sauce recipes)

Combine all ingredients and fill pancakes.

Toreador Pancakes

1 small onion, chopped
1 tablespoon butter
½ pound corned beef, chopped
½ pound tomatoes *or* 1 can tomatoes
salt and pepper
crushed potato chips

1. Fry onion in butter and mix in chopped corned beef.
2. Make pancakes and fill with corned beef mixture.
3. Peel fresh tomatoes and purée with salt and pepper or purée canned tomatoes.
4. Put pancakes in heatproof dish. Pour tomato purée over. Sprinkle with crushed potato chips and reheat.

SWEET PANCAKES

Pancake batter (as above)

Fillings

Mandarin Cream

½ cup heavy cream
2 large oranges *or* 3 mandarin oranges
juice of 1 orange

1. Whip cream, combine with orange segments.
2. Fill pancakes and roll up.
3. Warm orange juice and pour over.

Cottage Cheese and Pineapple

½ pound cottage cheese
6 tablespoons chopped fresh pineapple
pineapple juice

1. Combine cottage cheese and pineapple. Fill pancake and roll up.
2. Heat pineapple juice and pour over.

Banana Cream

4 large bananas, mashed
½ cup heavy cream
½ teaspoon nutmeg

Combine all ingredients and fill pancakes.

PANCAKES, AMERICAN STYLE or DROP SCONES

1¼ cups flour (whole-meal)
2½ teaspoons baking powder
¾ teaspoon salt
1 egg
1¼ cups milk
3 tablespoons melted fat

1. Place a griddle over low heat to warm.
2. Sift flour, baking powder, and salt into a bowl.
3. Beat egg and add milk and fat to it. Slowly stir this into the flour mixture, mixing only until the dry ingredients are wet.
4. When the griddle is hot enough to make a drop of cold water dance, grease it. Drop the batter from a large spoon lightly spreading with the back of the spoon to about 4 inches in diameter.
5. Cook over low heat until golden brown. Turn and brown the other side. Remove and stack.

Serve with bacon, eggs, ham, stewed or fresh fruit, or any of the fillings previously suggested in this section.

WAFFLES

1 cup whole-meal flour
1 egg
small amount of melted butter
½ cup milk
small amount of melted lard

1. Make the batter by beating flour, egg, butter, and milk together.
2. Clean, heat, and grease both compartments of the waffle iron with melted lard. Reheat until fat is hot.
3. Pour batter from a jug into one side of the iron, clamp other side over, and cook for 4 to 5 minutes (or according to the manufacturer's instructions).
4. Turn out and serve hot.

Serve with any stewed or fresh fruit and cream, or with fillings previously suggested in this section.

Salads, Salad Dressings, and Relishes

All regular salad vegetables are suitable, but some variations in the salad dressings may be necessary.

Four basic recipes have been included. These may be varied by the addition of any other ingredients that do not contain sugar or white flour.

Some basic recipes for side salads and relishes are also included.

These salads may be served with any cold meat or fish, including salami, liver sausage, etc.

Some recipes such as meat loaf will need to be adapted (see Meat recipes).

Bran may be added to any salad without affecting the taste in any way.

FRENCH DRESSING

3 tablespoons olive or other salad oil
1 tablespoon herb-flavored or wine vinegar
½ teaspoon dry mustard
½ teaspoon salt
freshly ground black pepper
1 crushed clove of garlic
1 tablespoon chopped fresh herbs (optional)

Combine all the ingredients.

Larger quantities of French Dressing may be prepared and stored in a screw-top jar in the refrigerator for a few weeks.

MAYONNAISE

(Makes about ¾ cup mayonnaise.)

1 egg yolk
½ level teaspoon dry mustard
½ level teaspoon salt
¼ level teaspoon pepper
½ cup oil
1 tablespoon white vinegar

1. Allow all the ingredients to reach room temperature.
2. Mix the egg yolk with the mustard, salt, and pepper, then beat in the cup of oil *drop by drop.*
3. Continue adding the oil until the sauce becomes thick and creamy.
4. When all the oil has been added, add the vinegar gradually and mix thoroughly.

THOUSAND ISLAND MAYONNAISE

½ cup mayonnaise
1 tablespoon finely chopped stuffed olives
1 teaspoon finely chopped onion
1 egg, hard-boiled and chopped
1 tablespoon finely chopped sweet green pepper
1 teaspoon chopped parsley
1 level teaspoon tomato paste

Mix all the ingredients together until evenly combined. Leave mayonnaise to stand for at least 30 minutes before serving to allow flavors to combine.

YOGURT DRESSING

½ cup natural yogurt
2 tablespoons fresh light cream
3 teaspoons lemon juice
salt and pepper

1. Pour yogurt into a bowl. Beat in cream and lemon juice. Season.
2. Leave in cool place for 15 minutes before using.

Variations

Add 2 finely chopped, hard-boiled eggs and 1 ounce of finely chopped anchovy fillets.

Add 2 level teaspoons curry powder and 1 level tablespoon relish (see recipe).

COLESLAW

3 to 4 cups shredded red or white cabbage
1 apple
1 large carrot
½ onion
salt and pepper
1 ounce peanuts
1 cup plain yogurt

1. Shred cabbage. Grate apple, carrot, and onion.
2. Add seasoning and peanuts.
3. Combine with yogurt.

Serve with any cold meat.

CELERY and TOMATO SALAD

3 slices bacon
3 thick slices of whole-meal bread
¼ cup margarine
½ teaspoon (level) mixed fresh or dried herbs (parsley, sage, rosemary, bay leaf, thyme, etc.)
4 large tomatoes
4 sticks of celery
2 medium-sized carrots

Dressing

1 tablespoon lemon juice
2 tablespoons oil
¼ level teaspoon salt
pinch of mustard
pepper

1. Cut bacon into small pieces. Remove crusts from bread, cut bread into ½-inch cubes.
2. Place bacon in a small saucepan over a low heat and fry slowly until crisp and golden brown. Remove from saucepan and drain on paper towel.
3. Add margarine to fat remaining in saucepan; heat until melted. Add dried herbs and bread cubes, fry, stirring occasionally, until golden brown and crisp. Drain on paper towels.

4. Place tomatoes in a bowl and cover with boiling water. Let stand for 1 minute, drain, then peel and chop.
5. Wash and slice celery. Wash, peel, and grate carrots.
6. Place lemon juice, oil, salt, mustard, and a dash of pepper in a serving bowl; beat with a fork.
7. Add tomatoes, celery, carrots, bacon, and fried bread. Stir mixture carefully, until coated with dressing.

Serve within 2 hours.

RICE SALAD

1 cup long grain Brown Rice
French Dressing (see recipe)
cooked peas, corn, sweet peppers
celery, apple, walnut pieces

1. Cook rice in boiling salted water (as directed in Rice and Pasta section). Drain and cool.
2. Mix French Dressing.
3. Toss all ingredients together.

Serve as a side salad.

SALADE NIÇOISE

1½ cups shredded ham, flaked tuna fish, chicken, or shrimp
1½ cups of any cooked green vegetable, e.g., peas, string beans, etc.
mixed chopped herbs
½ cucumber
4 tomatoes, thinly sliced
anchovy fillets and black olives
French Dressing (see recipe)

1. Put the meat or fish in a salad bowl.
2. Put the vegetables on top, then the herbs, sliced cucumber, and last the sliced tomatoes.
3. Arrange anchovy fillets and olives on top in a lattice design.
4. Add French Dressing.

Serve with thin slices of whole-meal bread and butter.

APPLE and MINT RELISH

1 large apple
2 tablespoons apricot purée (made from dried apricots)
1 tablespoon vinegar
1 tablespoon chopped mint
salt and cayenne

Peel and grate the apple coarsely. Mix at once with the rest of the ingredients. The mixture should be both sharp and sweet.

MUSTARD RELISH

2 pounds small onions
2 pounds mixed vegetables (cauliflower, green tomatoes, zucchini, cucumber)
salt
2 ounces dry mustard
½ cup whole-meal flour
½ ounce turmeric
5 cups vinegar

1. Dice the vegetables into small pieces. Place in an earthenware dish and sprinkle with salt. Let stand for 12 hours.
2. Put the mustard, flour, and turmeric in a small dish and add a little vinegar. Mix to a smooth paste.
3. Wash the salt from the vegetables. Put the vegetables into a pan with the rest of the vinegar. Bring to a boil and simmer for 20 minutes.
4. Add the mustard paste, stirring continuously until the mixture has thickened. Simmer for another 5 minutes, stirring occasionally. Cool.
5. Pour into warmed jars and cover.

Brown Rice and Whole-meal Pasta

These are easy to cook although they take a little longer than regular rice and pasta. The texture is firm and the flavor slightly nutty.

They can be substituted into any regular recipe as long as extra time is allowed for cooking. Some examples of this are given along with the basic recipes.

BROWN RICE

COOKING TIME: 35 MINUTES

4 cups water
salt
1 cup long-grain brown rice (for 2 portions)

1. Bring the water to a boil and add the salt.
2. Add the rice slowly, keeping it boiling, and cook for 35 minutes.
3. Drain and wash with hot water.

Serve with main meals, or cool and use as a base for salad (see Salad section).

PASTA

COOKING TIME: 12 TO 15 MINUTES

2 cups water (a portion)
salt
macaroni or whole-meal spaghetti (allow 2 ounces a portion)

1. Bring the water to a boil and add the salt.
2. Drop macaroni into the water or hold the spaghetti and push gently into the water until it softens and is completely covered.

3. Boil for 12 to 15 minutes, then test the pasta—it should be tender, so be careful not to overcook it.
4. Drain and serve immediately.

Serve as a main meal with a Bolognese, Neapolitan, or cheese sauce. Any of these may be easily adapted from the regular recipe by omitting sugar and substituting whole-meal for regular flour.

BAKED MACARONI

OVEN TEMPERATURE: 350°F
COOKING TIME: 30 MINUTES

- 6 ounces (1½ cups) whole-meal macaroni
- salt
- 6 ounces (1½ cups) cheese (grated)
- 2 eggs
- ¾ pint (2 cups) milk
- salt and pepper
- 2 tomatoes

Boil macaroni in salted water for 10 minutes. Drain. Grease an oven-proof dish well. Put macaroni and cheese in layers in dish. Beat eggs, milk, and seasoning together. Pour over macaroni. Sprinkle with grated cheese and decorate with sliced tomatoes. Bake at 350°F for 30 minutes.

CANNELLONI

OVEN TEMPERATURE: 400°F
COOKING TIME: 7 TO 10 MINUTES

Batter
- 4 ounces whole-meal flour (1 cup)
- 1 egg
- 1 egg yolk
- 1 tablespoon melted butter
- salt and pepper

Filling
- 1 pound spinach
- ¼ cup milk or cream cheese
- salt and pepper
- cheese or Mornay Sauce (see Eggs Mollet Florentine)

1. Prepare batter as for pancakes. Let stand for ½ hour. Fry small flat pancakes, stack them, and set aside.
2. Cook the spinach in boiling water for 5 minutes. Drain. Chop and mix in milk or cheese and seasoning.
3. Fill pancakes with this mixture, roll up, and arrange in a greased ovenproof dish.
4. Make cheese sauce. Pour over the cannelloni and brown in a hot oven for 7 to 10 minutes.

FRIED RICE SPECIAL

COOKING TIME: 40 MINUTES

- 2 medium-sized onions
- 2 tablespoons oil
- 1½ cups long-grain brown rice
- salt and pepper
- ½ level teaspoon turmeric
- 2½ cups chicken stock
- ¼ pound mushrooms
- small package frozen corn
- 1 cup shelled almonds
- ½ cup white raisins

1. Peel and finely chop onions. Place half the oil in large frying pan. Add onions and fry gently for 5 minutes, without browning. Add rice, salt, pepper, and turmeric. Fry gently, stirring for about 5 minutes. Reduce heat, add cold stock, cover with lid, and simmer for 35 minutes, stirring occasionally.
2. Quarter the mushrooms. Cook corn in boiling salted water. Place almonds in a small bowl, cover with boiling water, and let stand for 1 minute; drain, remove skins, and split lengthwise. Heat rest of oil in frying pan, add almonds, and fry gently for 5 minutes until golden brown. Drain.
3. Add mushrooms, raisins, corn, and half the almonds to rice. Stir well, cover, and continue to cook for 5 minutes until rice is tender.
4. Place rice on warm serving dish and sprinkle the remaining almonds over it.

DANISH RISOTTO

COOKING TIME: 1 HOUR

- ¼ cup butter
- 1½ cups chopped onion
- 1 stalk celery, chopped
- 1 green pepper, cleaned and sliced
- 1 cup Brown Rice
- 2½ cups ham stock
- ½ cup seedless raisins
- 1 teaspoon (level) salt
- ¼ teaspoon (level) pepper
- 1 cup chopped pineapple (fresh)
- 1 cup sliced peaches (fresh)
- 8 ounces cooked ham, cut into cubes

1. Melt the butter in a heavy saucepan and cook the onion, celery, and pepper without browning.
2. Add the rice and cook for 3 to 4 minutes until the rice has absorbed all the butter and is slightly brown.
3. Pour in 2 cups of the stock, add the raisins and seasoning and cook for 20 minutes, stirring occasionally.
4. Add the fruit and ham and the rest of the stock. Continue cooking until the rice is cooked and the stock has been absorbed.

Serve with a green salad.

N.B. Other fruit, e.g., apple and orange may be used in place of the pineapple and peaches.

Desserts

Use as much and as many varieties of fresh fruit as you like. Frozen or canned fruits may be used in any of the recipes given here, as long as no sugar or syrup has been added to them. You may like to can your own fruit; if so, any normal method of canning can be used, but, of course, you must not add any sugar during the canning process.

Many of the recipes may be adapted by using other fruits that may be available. Don't be afraid to experiment! Purèed bananas, apricots, peaches, dried apples, and other dried fruits, unsweetened orange and pineapple juices, etc., can all be used to give natural sweetness to any recipes you adapt or invent.

COLD DESSERTS

NO COOKING

FRESH FRUIT SALAD

3 pounds ripe fruit, e.g., melon, oranges, dessert pears, bananas, grapes, plums, etc.
1 cup of water
½ cup of unsweetened orange juice
½ cup of unsweetened pineapple juice

1. Wash and prepare the fruit, then dice into even-sized pieces.
2. Mix the water and fruit juices together, then pour the mixture over the diced fruit.
3. Allow the fruit salad to stand for approximately 1 hour before serving, so that the flavors of the fruits can merge.

Serve with plenty of whipped cream.

Variations

Use different kinds and amounts of fruits for variety.

Add a tablespoon of chopped nuts to the salad to give it an interesting texture.

AVOCADO COCKTAIL

2 avocados, peeled and pitted
lemon juice
1 cup seeded, halved grapes
½ cup sliced peaches
½ cup strawberries
1 cup water
sour cream

1. Cut the avocados into cubes and add some lemon juice to prevent discoloration.
2. Combine with the rest of the ingredients.

Serve in individual glasses, topped with sour cream.

ORANGE CHEESECAKE

3 oranges
1 lemon
2 tablespoons gelatin
2 eggs
1 cup milk
3 cups cottage cheese
½ cup heavy cream

For the cheesecake topping:

2 tablespoons butter
1 cup whole-meal bread crumbs

1. Grate the rind of two oranges and squeeze the juice from all three. Add the juice from the lemon. Place 4 tablespoons of orange juice in a small bowl and sprinkle the gelatin on top.
2. Beat the egg yolks and milk together lightly. Heat gently, but do not boil. Add the moist gelatin and stir until dissolved. Cool until nearly set, then add the orange rind and 6 tablespoons orange juice.
3. Mix together the cheese and gelatin mixture.
4. Beat the egg whites until stiff.
5. Beat the cream until stiff.
6. Fold the cream and egg whites into the cheese mixture.
7. Turn into a waxed-paper-lined 8-inch pan.
8. Melt the butter, then add the bread crumbs. Press waxed-paper-topping firmly down into the cheese mixture.
9. Chill well, then take the cheesecake out of the pan and pull off the lining paper. Decorate with orange segments and whipped cream.

Variations

Use apricot purée and apricot halves as a flavoring instead of oranges.
Use peaches as a flavoring instead of oranges.

ORANGE MOUSSE

1 tablespoon gelatin
½ cup lukewarm water
1 egg
2 tablespoons powdered milk
2 cups unsweetened orange juice (canned, fresh, or frozen)
grated orange rind

1. Put gelatin into a cup with 2 tablespoons of cold water. Warm the cup in a saucepan of simmering water and stir to dissolve the gelatin.
2. Separate the egg.
3. Beat the ½ cup lukewarm water, egg yolk, powdered milk, orange juice, orange rind, and gelatin together. Let mixture stand in a cool place until it is ready to jell.
4. Beat the egg white until stiff, then fold it into the mixture.
5. Pour the mixture into a jello mold and refrigerate until firm. Turn out and serve decorated with fresh grapes or orange segments.

SUMMER PUDDING

- 6 large slices whole-meal bread
- 1½ pounds soft fruit (rhubarb, raspberries, strawberries, gooseberries, black or red currants, blueberries, pitted cherries, or a mixture of fruits)
- 5 tablespoons water

1. Remove crusts from bread, cut into strips, and line base and sides of a 1-quart pudding pan. Save enough to make a cover.
2. Simmer fruit and water for about 10 minutes.
3. Put hot fruit into bread-lined pan and cover with bread.
4. Cover with a plate and put a heavy weight on top.
5. Refrigerate overnight.
6. Turn out on to plate.

Serve with whipped cream.

BANANA SNOW

- 6 medium bananas
- 3 tablespoons lemon juice
- 1 cup natural yogurt
- 1 cup heavy cream
- whites of 2 eggs

1. Mash bananas to a purée with lemon juice. Stir in yogurt and mix well.
2. Whip cream until lightly stiff. Beat egg whites.
3. Fold cream and egg whites alternately into banana mixture. Turn into serving dish. Chill thoroughly before serving.

FRUIT FOOL

- 1 pound fruit (gooseberries, apples, black or red currants, rhubarb, blueberries, raspberries, etc.)
- 3 tablespoons water
- 1 cup heavy cream

1. Wash and prepare fruit. Put in pan with water. Bring slowly to boil, cover and simmer until soft. Remove from heat.
2. Purée in an electric blender. Let stand until completely cold.
3. Whip cream until lightly stiff and gradually fold in the fruit purée.
4. Place in individual dishes and chill.

Serve with whipped cream shaped into whirls on top and sprinkled with nuts.

BANANA ICE CREAM

1 small can evaporated milk (approx. 1 cup)
2 eggs
3 ripe bananas

1. Place the unopened can of milk in a saucepan of boiling water and boil for 15 minutes.
2. Cool, then chill the can for several hours.
3. Open the can, pour the milk into a large bowl and whip the milk until it has tripled in volume.
4. Separate the eggs and beat the egg whites until stiff.
5. Mash the bananas, then add the bananas and the egg yolks to the whipped milk.
6. Gently mix in the whipped egg whites, so that they are evenly distributed through the banana mixture.
7. Pour into a freezer container and freeze until firm.

Serve plain or with more chopped bananas and fresh cream.

HOT DESSERTS

FALL PIE

COOKING TIME: 50 MINUTES
OVEN TEMPERATURE: 20 MINUTES AT 425°F
30 MINUTES AT 375°F

Pastry
½ cup (generous) lard or other shortening
2 tablespoons cold water
salt
2 cups whole-meal flour
2 teaspoons baking powder

Filling
1 pound prunes
1 pound plums
¾ cup liquid (see step 3)

1. Pour enough water over the prunes to cover them, then soak them overnight.
2. Make up the American Pie Pastry (see Pastry section).
3. Drain the prunes and plums and put into a pie dish. Add ¾ cup of liquid. This may be the liquid used in soaking the prunes, weak tea or water, or a mixture of these.
4. Roll out the pastry and cover the pie. Bake for 20 minutes at 425°F, then 30 minutes at 375°F.

Serve with whipped cream.

Variations
Use different proportions and types of fruit in the pie.
Add some blanched almonds to the fruit.

GRILLED CINNAMON PEACHES

COOKING TIME: 10 MINUTES

fresh peaches (1 per person)
ground cinnamon

1. Halve the peaches and remove pits.
2. Sprinkle liberally with cinnamon.
3. Arrange in ovenproof dish and bake gently until peaches are just soft and heated through.

Serve with whipped cream.

FRUIT CRUMBLE

COOKING TIME: 1 HOUR
OVEN TEMPERATURE: 375°F, LOWER TO 350°F AFTER 15 MINUTES

1 pound fruit, e.g., apples, rhubarb, gooseberries, blueberries, plums, red or black currants, etc.
3 tablespoons butter or other shortening
1½ cups whole-meal flour

1. Wash and prepare the fruit, then place it in an ovenproof dish.
2. Blend the butter or shortening with the flour.
3. Sprinkle the crumble mixture evenly over the fruit. Press down lightly.
4. Bake in the oven for 15 minutes at 375°F, then 45 minutes at 350°F.

Serve with fresh or sour cream.

APPLE CHARLOTTE

COOKING TIME: 1 HOUR
OVEN TEMPERATURE: 350°F

1½ cups whole-meal bread crumbs
4 ounces butter
rind and juice of 1 lemon
1 pound apples

1. Mix together the bread crumbs, butter, and a little grated lemon rind.
2. Peel core, and slice the apples. Place the apples in a greased ovenproof dish in alternate layers with the bread-crumb mixture. Sprinkle each layer of apple slices with a little lemon juice and rind.
3. Finish the layers with a layer of bread crumbs.
4. Bake at 350°F for 1 hour.

Serve with fresh cream, sour cream, or custard sauce (see Sauces section).

Variation: Use any fruit in place of apples.

DATE and ORANGE FLAN

COOKING TIME: 20 TO 30 MINUTES
OVEN TEMPERATURE: 375°F

- Shortcrust, or Pie, Pastry (see Pastry recipes)
- 1½ cups chopped pitted dates
- 3 medium-sized oranges, peeled and cut
- ½ cup water

1. Make pastry. Roll out thinly and line greased 6-inch flan pan. Bake without filling at 375°F for 20 to 30 minutes.
2. Put dates, oranges, and water in saucepan and heat gently until dates are soft and water has been absorbed. Let stand until cool.
3. When flan crust and mixture are cool, put mixture into crust and let stand to set.

Serve with whipped cream, orange slices and segments, and nuts.

Cakes and Cookies

Home baking is rapidly becoming a dying art. Our forebears used to do all their own baking while we, nowadays, rely almost completely upon large manufacturers to produce our cakes and cookies. Virtually all of these regular convenience foods are very refined and so are totally unsuitable.

Go back to the good old days! Bring out the baking pans and have a go at these recipes. You will be surprised by the results!

BANANA NUT LOAF

COOKING TIME: 1¼ HOURS
OVEN TEMPERATURE: 350°F

- 1 cup water
- ½ cup cooking oil
- 2 eggs, beaten
- 2 cups whole-meal flour
- 4 teaspoons (heaping) baking powder
- grated rind of 1 lemon
- 1 large ripe banana, mashed to a pulp
- 1 cup chopped mixed nuts
- 1 cup white raisins
- dash of salt

1. Mix together the water, oil, and eggs.
2. Mix all the dry ingredients together, then stir the dry ingredients and the banana pulp alternately into the liquid mixture. Beat until smooth.
3. Pour mixture into well-greased cake or loaf pan and bake at 350°F for 1¼ hours. Let stand to cool for 5 minutes before removing from the pan.

FRUIT and NUT LOAF

COOKING TIME: 1 HOUR
OVEN TEMPERATURE: 325°F

- 1 cup (generous) whole-meal flour
- dash of salt
- 2 teaspoons baking powder
- 1 teaspoon cinnamon
- ½ teaspoon mixed spice
- 2 tablespoons butter
- 1 grated apple
- 1 egg, well beaten
- 4 tablespoons milk
- ¾ cup chopped dates
- ½ cup chopped walnuts
- 2 teaspoons grated orange rind

1. Mix the flour, salt, baking powder, and spices together.
2. Cream the butter with a little flour and then add the grated apple.
3. Slowly add the egg and the milk. Beat the mixture well.
4. Fold in the remaining fruit and nuts, then spoon the mixture into a greased cake pan.
5. Bake at 325°F for approximately 1 hour. Let the cake stand in the pan for 5 minutes before turning it onto a wire rack.

Serve plain or with butter.

APPLE LOAF

COOKING TIME: 1 HOUR
OVEN TEMPERATURE: 350°F

- 3 cups whole-meal flour
- 3 teaspoons baking powder
- dash of salt
- ½ teaspoon nutmeg
- ½ teaspoon mixed spice
- 3 tablespoons butter
- 4 apples, peeled and cored
- 1 cup raisins (dark or white)
- ½ cup blanched almonds or brazil nuts
- 1 egg, beaten
- finely grated rind and juice of 1 lemon
- milk to mix
- 2 tablespoons flaked almonds, for the topping

1. Mix the flour, baking powder, salt, and spices together. Blend the butter with the flour.
2. Dice the apples, then add the apple, dried fruit, and nuts to the mixture.
3. Stir in the egg, lemon rind and juice. Stir in enough milk to give a sticky consistency.
4. Grease a loaf pan, then spoon the mixture into the pan. Smooth the mixture to make even, then sprinkle the flaked almonds over the top.
5. Bake for approximately 1 hour at 350°F. Take the loaf out of the pan carefully.

APPLE SHORTCAKE

COOKING TIME: 30 TO 35 MINUTES
OVEN TEMPERATURE: 350°F

- ½ cup butter
- 2 cups whole-meal flour
- 1 egg
- 1 teaspoon baking powder
- dash of salt
- grated rind and juice of half a lemon
- 3 apples, peeled and coarsely grated
- ½ cup chopped dates

1. Cream the butter with a little of the flour until smooth. Add the egg and beat well.
2. Mix in the flour, baking powder, salt, lemon rind and lemon juice. The mixture should hold together in a dough at this stage.
3. Divide the mixture in two. Press half the mixture into a greased 8-inch cake pan.
4. Spread with grated apples and dates. Cover with the remaining dough and press lightly down.
5. Bake at 350°F for 30 to 35 minutes.

DATE SHORTBREAD

COOKING TIME: 20 TO 30 MINUTES
OVEN TEMPERATURE: 300°F

- 3 tablespoons butter
- 1 cup chopped dates
- 1 cup (generous) whole-meal flour

1. Melt the butter. Let the chopped dates stand in the butter for 2 to 3 minutes.
2. Add the flour. Mix well, then pack into a pan.
3. Bake at 300°F for 20 to 30 minutes.

NUTTIES

COOKING TIME: 30 TO 40 MINUTES
OVEN TEMPERATURE: 350°F

- ½ cup butter
- 2 cups rolled oats
- ½ cup chopped peanuts
- ½ cup raisins (white or dark)
- 1 large egg, beaten

1. Melt the butter. Add the dry ingredients and the beaten egg and mix well.
2. Spread into a shallow pan and bake at 350°F for 30 to 40 minutes.

APRICOT OATIES

COOKING TIME: 25 MINUTES
OVEN TEMPERATURE: 375°F

- 2 cups dried apricots
- 1½ cups rolled oats
- 1 cup whole-meal flour
- 2 teaspoons baking powder
- ½ cup shortening
- 1 egg

1. Preheat the oven to 375°F.
2. Grease a shallow 7-inch square baking pan.
3. Put apricots in a saucepan with water. Bring to a boil and cook gently, stirring occasionally until all the water has been absorbed and the apricots are tender.
4. Take one-fourth of the apricots and purée them.
5. Mix the rolled oats, flour, and baking powder together. Add the shortening. Blend the shortening with the dry ingredients.
6. Add the beaten egg and the puréed apricots. Mix well.
7. Press half the oat mixture into the pan. Spread the remaining whole apricots over this, then top with the remaining oat mixture. Press down lightly.
8. Bake at 375°F for 25 minutes.
9. Let stand to cool in the pan, then cut into squares.

RAISIN and APPLE SLICE

COOKING TIME: 30 MINUTES
OVEN TEMPERATURE: 450°F

Flaky Pastry (see Pastry recipes)
- 2 cups whole-meal flour
- salt
- 2 teaspoons baking powder
- ⅓ cup shortening
- ⅓ cup butter
- a few drops of lemon juice
- water to mix

Filling
- ½ cup white raisins
- 3 apples
- lemon juice
- cinnamon
- 1 egg, beaten

1. Make up Flaky Pastry. After final chilling, roll out into an oblong ¼-½ inch thick. Score 1 inch from the edges to make a border.
2. Fill the oblong with the raisins.
3. Quarter, core, and slice the apples. Arrange in layers on top of the raisins.
4. Sprinkle with lemon juice and cinnamon.
5. Brush generously with egg and bake.

Serve with cream or puréed fruit sauce.

Variations

Other fruit may be used in place of apple.

Use with a filling of ground beef topped with tomato/onion/mushrooms, etc.

APPLE and RAISIN CAKE

COOKING TIME: 45 MINUTES
OVEN TEMPERATURE: 375°F

- 2 cups whole-meal flour
- 2 teaspoons baking powder
- dash of salt
- 2 tablespoons shortening
- 1½ cups raisins
- grated rind of 1 lemon
- 4 medium apples
- 1 egg, beaten
- 3 tablespoons milk

1. Mix flour, baking powder, and salt. Break up the shortening into small pieces, then blend it with the flour.
2. Stir in the raisins and lemon rind.
3. Peel, core, then finely chop the apples. Add the apples, egg, and the milk to the mixture and mix well.
4. Place the mixture in a greased cake pan and bake at 375°F for 45 minutes.
5. When baked, take out and place on a greased wire rack to cool.

RHUBARB and DATE CAKE

COOKING TIME: 1 TO 1½ HOURS
OVEN TEMPERATURE: 375°F

- ½ cup shortening
- 2 cups whole-meal flour
- 3 teaspoons baking powder
- ½ pound rhubarb
- 1½ cups chopped dates
- 1 large egg, beaten
- 4 tablespoons milk

1. Blend shortening with the flour and baking powder.
2. Chop the rhubarb into small cubes. Add the rhubarb and the dates to the mixture, and stir.
3. Add the egg and milk and mix well.
4. Pour the mixture into a cake pan and bake at 375°F for 1 to 1½ hours.

FRUIT COOKIES

COOKING TIME: 15 TO 20 MINUTES
OVEN TEMPERATURE: 350°F

- ½ cup shortening
- 2 cups whole-meal flour
- 1 egg yolk
- water to mix
- 1 cup white raisins
- almond or vanilla extract to taste (approx. 1 teaspoon) or grated orange rind, lemon extract, or cinnamon

1. Blend the shortening with the flour. Add the egg yolk and enough cold water to form a soft dough.
2. Add the fruit and the flavoring and knead the mixture lightly.
3. Roll the dough out on a floured board until it is ¼-½ inch thick. Cut the cookies out into any shapes you like.
4. Bake at 350°F for 15 to 20 minutes. Do *not* bake them until they are hard to the touch.

Breakfasts

Many foods regularly eaten at breakfast are acceptable without alteration. For example, unsweetened fruit juice, fresh fruit, ham, eggs, cheese, bacon, etc.

However, it will be necessary to modify any foods containing regular flour, for example, bread (see Bread recipes) and pancakes (see Pancake recipes).

Care must be taken in choosing breakfast cereals. Check the labels. The ones that say they are made from whole cereal and do not contain sugar are the best.

Of course, maple syrup and jelly should be avoided, and fresh stewed fruits used in their place.

Some suggestions for items you might like to try for breakfast are given in this section.

MUESLI I

NO COOKING

1 cup of bran
2 cups of rolled oats
1 cup of chopped mixed nuts
1 cup of mixed dried fruit
½ cup of dried apple flakes

Mix all the ingredients together, then store in an airtight jar until needed. Serve with fresh milk or yogurt.

Variations

Vary the quantities of each ingredient to suit your own taste.

Add dried grated orange peel to give the muesli an interesting orangy tang.

Add diced fresh fruit such as apples, bananas, or peaches to the muesli just before serving.

MUESLI II
(To serve immediately)

NO COOKING

- ¼ cup nuts (Brazils, walnuts, hazelnuts)
- 1 crisp eating apple
- 1 orange
- 1 cup plain yogurt
- 1½ cups rolled oats (natural oats)
- ½ cup bran (optional)
- ½ cup white raisins

1. Chop or coarsely grate the nuts.
2. Quarter the apple and remove the core, but do not peel. Chop it into small cubes.
3. Finely grate the peel of the orange.
4. Peel the orange, remove seeds and tough skin, and chop the fruit small.
5. Mix all the ingredients together. If possible leave in the refrigerator or a cool place for 1 hour before serving.

BRAN MUFFINS

COOKING TIME: 15 MINUTES
OVEN TEMPERATURE: 425°F

- 2 cups whole-meal flour
- 2 cups bran
- 5 level teaspoons baking powder
- 1 level teaspoon salt
- 2 eggs
- 2 cups milk
- 1 tablespoon oil
- 4 ounces dates, chopped (optional)

1. Put flour, bran, baking powder, and salt into a bowl. Mix well together.
2. Beat eggs, milk, and oil together.
3. Add egg mixture and dates (if used) to dry ingredients. Stir only enough to mix evenly.
4. Fill 20 greased deep muffin tins. Bake for approximately 15 minutes.

Serve fresh with butter and cream or cottage cheese.

FRENCH TOAST

COOKING TIME: 6 MINUTES

- 2 eggs
- salt and pepper (omit if serving with fruit)
- ⅔ cup milk
- 4 slices whole-meal bread

1. Beat the eggs together in a bowl. Season. Add milk and mix.
2. Dip slices of bread, one at a time, into the mixture until well soaked.
3. Fry in butter for about 3 minutes each side.

Serve with fried, fresh, or canned tomatoes or with fresh or stewed fruit.

KEDGEREE

COOKING TIME: 1 HOUR

- 1 cup Brown Rice
- ¼ cup butter
- 8 ounces cooked, flaked, smoked haddock
- 2 hard-boiled eggs, roughly chopped
- seasoning
- 1 egg, beaten
- 2 to 3 tablespoons cream

1. Boil the rice until tender (approx. 40 minutes), drain well.
2. Melt the butter in a frying pan. Add the fish and shake over the heat until hot.
3. Add the rice and chopped eggs. Season. Shake and stir well.
4. When very hot, add the egg and the cream. Quickly stir the mixture with a fork until cooked.
5. Turn out and serve immediately, garnished with parsley and lemon wedges.

Snacks

Whole-meal bread and biscuits can be used just as easily as regular bread and biscuits. It is the accompaniments, such as fruit, vegetables, eggs, meat, fish, and cheese, that matter and provide the interest and variety.

Bran may be added to "sandwiches" by sprinkling it on the buttered bread before the filling.

TOASTED SANDWICHES

Allow two slices of whole-meal bread per portion. If the filling is to be hot, prepare this beforehand. Sandwich together the filling and bread, and toast on both sides. Serve immediately on a hot plate. Garnish with watercress, parsley, tomatoes, etc.

Cold fillings

Sliced roast beef, mustard, and tomatoes.
Flaked salmon or tuna with cucumber and mayonnaise (see Salads).
Sliced Cheddar cheese with relishes (see Salads).

Hot fillings

Bacon and fried apple rings.
Scrambled egg, seasoning, and sliced cooked mushrooms.
Fried fillets of fish with tartare sauce (see Sauces).
Diced chicken and curry sauce (see Sauces).

CLUB SANDWICHES

Allow 3 slices of buttered whole-meal bread per person. If the filling is to be hot, prepare this beforehand. Layer the slices of bread with fillings. Toast and serve immediately. Garnish with olives and gherkins.

Fillings

1. Crisp lettuce and fresh pineapple ring.	1st layer
Cottage cheese and mild mustard.	2nd layer
2. Lettuce, sliced hard-boiled eggs, mayonnaise (see Salads).	1st layer
2 slices cheese and sliced tomato.	2nd layer
3. Sliced ham and raw onion rings.	1st layer
Seasoned scrambled egg.	2nd layer
4. Flaked salmon.	1st layer
Whipped butter and chopped gherkins.	2nd layer

OPEN SANDWICHES

Use thinly sliced whole-meal bread, pumpernickel or whole-meal crisp bread, e.g., Ry-Krisp. Butter well and serve on flat serving tray.

Toppings

Lettuce, peeled cooked shrimp, and mayonnaise (see Salads).
Sliced beef, natural yogurt, and sliced carrot.
Sliced salami and raw onion rings.
Smoked ham, prunes, and cottage cheese.
Sliced Camembert with fresh fruit.
Sliced Danish blue cheese with grapes.
Scrambled egg and anchovy fillets.

Garnish with parsley, watercress, and radish.

PLOWMAN'S LUNCH

whole-meal bread rolls
butter
cheese
relishes (see Salads)

Serve bread, butter, and large slice of cheese on a plate with relishes. *Garnish* with tomato, lettuce, and raw onion.

BROILED AVOCADO

8 strips bacon
4 whole-meal bread rolls
1 avocado, thinly sliced
mustard
2 cups grated cheese

1. Fry bacon, drain, and keep warm.
2. Split rolls, toast them and butter.
3. Top each half roll with avocado slices.
4. Brush with mustard.
5. Sprinkle with grated cheese, making sure avocado is completely covered.

Place under broiler until cheese melts. Top with bacon strips and serve immediately.

CHEESE AND APPLE TOASTS

4 slices whole-meal bread
a little butter
4 slices cheese, Gruyère or Cheddar
1 large eating apple
8 thin lean bacon slices

1. Toast the bread and spread with butter.
2. Top with cheese and toast for 1 minute under broiler.
3. Core the apple and cut into 8 segments. Roll a slice of bacon around a segment of apple.
4. Put two bacon rolls on each cheese toast and broil until bacon is crisp.
5. Garnish with a lettuce leaf, or watercress, or a tomato slice, and serve when piping hot.

BAKED STUFFED POTATOES

6 baked potatoes
salt and pepper to taste
¼ cup sour cream *or* 3 ounces cream cheese
1 cup chopped cucumber
1 egg, beaten (optional)
1 large eating apple
8 thin lean bacon slices

1. Cut potatoes in half lengthwise.
2. Scoop out, mash, and season.
3. Blend sour cream or cream cheese and cucumber into potato. If using egg, blend into mixture.
4. Fill potatoes.
5. Top with bacon rolls (see step 4 in previous recipe).

Potatoes may be prepared ahead of time, covered, and stored in refrigerator or may be wrapped in foil and frozen for a few weeks. Reheat for 20 to 30 minutes in 350°F oven.

Alternative Fillings

Corn and cheese.	Mash potato with seasoning, grated American or Cheddar cheese, and yogurt. Top with corn.
Cheese and bacon.	Mash potato with sliced Danish blue cheese, mayonnaise (see Salads), and parsley. Top with rasher of fried bacon.
Eggs and potatoes.	Mash potato with seasoning, butter, chopped hard-boiled egg whites. Top with sliced egg yolks, paprika, and chopped gherkins.
Farmhouse potatoes.	Mash potato with seasoning and a little cream cheese. Top with sliced cooked mushrooms and tomatoes, and a spoonful of scrambled egg.

Party Foods

The recipes in this section provide you with just a few ideas for parties, and should stimulate your imagination.

It is best to steer away from the "sweet" foods and make do with more interesting "savories." (Savories in recipes refer to "non-sweet," usually highly seasoned foods served at the end of a meal or as an appetizer.) A good general rule: Foods that can be eaten with regular bread and biscuits go just as well with whole-meal.

Use fruit and vegetables to give exciting color and interesting tastes.

CHEESE FONDUE

- 1 clove garlic
- 2 wineglasses dry white wine
- 4 cups grated Gruyère cheese
- 2 teaspoons whole-meal flour
- 1 tablespoon butter
- white pepper, grated nutmeg, paprika

1. Rub inside fondue pot with cut garlic.
2. Add wine and heat for 1 minute.

3. Add cheese and stir over medium heat until fondue thickens.
4. Mix flour with a little milk and add to the mixture.
5. Add butter and stir until melted.
6. Season to taste.

Serve with cubes of whole-meal bread and a green salad.

Variations

Sauté 1 pound button mushrooms in butter and add this to the mixture.

Add ½ teaspoon chopped tarragon, 1 teaspoon chopped parsley, pinch nutmeg, pinch black pepper.

Try a meat fondue.

CHEESE DIP

- 1 pound cottage cheese
- ⅔ cup sour cream
- 1 tablespoon lemon juice
- 2 to 3 tablespoons mayonnaise (see Salads)

1. Mix all the ingredients together.
2. Season to taste.
3. Garnish with paprika or chopped chives.

Serve with sticks of carrot or celery, scallions, chicory, radishes, or small crisp whole-meal biscuits or crisp breads, potato chips, etc.

Variations

Add small can crabmeat, extra lemon juice, and cucumber.

Add chopped chives, parsley, and crushed garlic.

Add 1 cup small raw mushrooms, ½ cup chopped cucumber, and small portion raw cauliflower.

Substitute flaked salmon for the cottage cheese, flavor with chili sauce, chopped gherkins, and capers.

Substitute mashed avocado for the cottage cheese, flavor with chopped onions and tomato.

COCKTAIL SAVORIES

CHEESE PASTRIES

Use to make cheese straws, cheese twists, tartlets, cocktail quiches.

SAVORY CHOUX BUNS (for recipe, see Pastry section)

Treat as regular pastry shells (vol-au-vents).

Filling 1

- 1 cup minced ham
- 1 teaspoon curry powder
- 1 tablespoon chutney
- ½ tablespoon shredded coconut
- 1 tablespoon white raisins

Filling 2

- 1 avocado
- 1 tablespoon lemon juice
- 1 tablespoon mayonnaise (see Salads)
- 2 tablespoons soft cream cheese

Also try a white sauce (see Sauces) with either mushrooms or shrimp, etc.

ASPARAGUS ROLLS

- 12 thin slices bread from small whole-meal loaf
- butter
- soft cream cheese or mayonnaise (see Salads)
- 12 cooked or canned asparagus

1. Cut crusts from bread.
2. Roll each slice with a rolling pin.
3. Spread with butter, then cheese (or mayonnaise).
4. Lay asparagus diagonally on the bread.
5. Roll so the asparagus tips show.

CANAPÉS

For the bases, use

- Toasted whole-meal bread
- Fried whole-meal bread
- Whole-meal Shortcrust Pastry (see Pastry section)
- Whole-meal biscuits

Cut into rounds, triangles, or other shapes.

Toppings

Mash sardines with chili sauce. Top with parsley.
Mash 2 egg yolks, ¼ cup butter, anchovy paste, seasoning.
Slices of Danish blue cheese topped with black grapes.
Rings of hard-boiled egg topped with caviar.

THINGS ON STICKS

Squares of cheese with grapes, or slices of fresh pineapple, or walnuts, or cocktail onions.

Scampi coated in seasoned whole-meal flour and deep fried.

Strips of fresh fish coated and friend as scampi.

Bacon rolls and tomato slices.

Squares of ham with fresh pineapple.

Drinks

Once again, fruits and fruit juices provide the best base for drinks. Coffee, tea, and cocoa are acceptable, provided, of course, you don't add sugar.

A few ideas for sweeter drinks are included; use these as a guide and invent some more for yourself.

BANANA MILK SHAKE

1	banana	per person
¾	cup of cold milk	

1. Mash the banana to a pulp.
2. Add the banana pulp to milk, then blend until the milk shake is thoroughly mixed.

Serve as soon as the milk shake is made. An ice cube can be added to each milk shake to make it really cold.

Variations: Flavor the milk shake with coffee, cocoa, or even cocoa and banana.

FRUITY FIZZ

1 cup unsweetened orange juice
1 cup unsweetened pineapple juice
2 cups soda water

Mix all the ingredients together.

Serve with ice.

Variations: Use any other mixture of fruit juices, for example, orange juice and apple juice; grapefruit juice and orange juice; pineapple juice and apple juice.

FRUIT CUP

1 lemon
1 orange
2 cups pineapple juice
1 cup orange juice
1 cup apple juice
1 cup grapefruit juice
1 cup water
sprig of mint

1. Slice the lemon and the orange into thin slices.
2. Mix all the fruit juices and the water together. Add the sliced fruit and the sprig of mint.

Serve well chilled. Add ice if you wish.

Variations: Vary the types and amounts of each of the fruit juices to suit your own taste.

ICED COFFEE

Make up strong coffee as usual. Pour the coffee over ice cubes.
Serve on its own, with milk or with slices of orange.

ICED TEA

Make up strong tea by pouring boiling water over a tea bag or a teaspoonful of tea leaves. Pour the tea over ice cubes. Strain if you use tea leaves.

Serve plain with milk, or with slices of lemon.

A selected bibliography

Aries, V. et al. Bacteria and the aetiology of cancer of the large bowel. The Journal of the British Society of Gastroenterology —Gut 10:34, 1969.

Bread: An assessment of the British bread industry. The TACC Report, Technology Assessment Consumerism Centre. London: Intermediate Publishing Limited, 1974.

Burkitt, D. P. Related disease—related cause? *The Lancet,* pp. 1229–1231, Dec. 6, 1969.

———. Relationship as a clue to causation. *The Lancet,* pp. 1237–1240, Dec. 12, 1970.

———. Possible relationships between bowel cancer and dietary habits. *Proceedings of the Royal Society of Medicine* 64:964, 1971.

———. The aetiology of appendicitis. *British Journal of Surgery* 58:695, 1971.

———. Epidemiology of cancer of the colon and rectum. *Cancer* 28:3, 1971.

———. Guest editorial: Some neglected leads to cancer causation. *Journal of the National Cancer Institute* 47:913, 1971.

———. Varicose veins, deep vein thrombosis, and haemorrhoids: epidemiology and suggested aetiology. *British Medical Journal* 2:556, 1972.

———. Effect of dietary fibre on stools and transit-times, and its role in the causation of disease. *The Lancet,* pp. 1408–1412, 1972.

———. Diseases of the alimentary tract and Western diets. *Proceedings 11th Conference International Society Geographic Pathology* 39:177, 1973.

———. Epidemiology of large bowel disease: the role of fibre. *Proceedings Nutrition Society* 32:145, 1973.

——— and James, P. A. Low-residue diets and hiatus hernia. *The Lancet,* pp. 128–130, 1973.

———. Some diseases characteristic of modern Western civilization: A possible common causative factor. *Clinical Radiology* 24:271, 1973.

———. Some diseases characteristic of modern Western civilization. *British Medical Journal* 1:274, 1973.

———; Walker, A. R. P.; and Painter, N. S. Dietary fiber and disease. *Journal of the American Medical Association* 229: 1068, 1974.

Cleave, T. L.: The neglect of natural principles in current medical practice. *Journal of the Royal Naval Medical Service* 42:55, 1956.

———. *Peptic Ulcer*. Bristol: Wright, 1962.

——— and Campbell, G. D. *Diabetes, Coronary Thrombosis, and the Saccharine Disease*. Bristol: Wright, 1966.

———. *The Saccharine Disease*. Bristol: Wright, 1974.

Crowther, J. S. et al. The effect of a chemically defined diet on the faecal flora and faecal steroid concentration. *The Journal of the British Society of Gastroenterology*–Gut 14:790, 1973.

Cummings, J. H. Progress report–Dietary Fibre. *The Journal of the British Society of Gastroenterology*–Gut 14:69, 1973.

Diet and Coronary Heart Disease. Report of the Advisory Panel of the Committee on Medical Aspects of Food Policy (Nutrition) on Diet in relation to Cardiovascular and Cerebrovascular Disease. London: Her Majesty's Stationery Office, 1974.

Drasar, B. S. et al. The relation between diet and the gut microflora in man. *Proceedings Nutrition Society* 32:49, 1973.

——— and Hill, M. J. Intestinal bacteria and cancer. *The American Journal of Clinical Nutrition* 25:1399, 1972.

——— and Irving, D. Environmental factors and cancer of the colon and breast. *British Journal Cancer* 27:167, 1973.

Eastwood, M. A. Dietary fibre in human nutrition. *Journal of the Science of Food and Agriculture* 25:1523, 1974.

——— and Terry, S. I. Diet and gastroenterology. *British Journal of Hospital Medicine,* November 1974.

——— and Mitchell, W. D. The place of vegetable fibre in diet. *British Journal of Hospital Medicine,* January 1974.

———. Vegetable fibre: its physical properties. *Proceedings Nutrition Society* 32:137, 1973.

———. Perspectives on the bran hypothesis. *The Lancet,* pp. 1029–1033, May 25, 1974.

Ershoff, B. H. Antitoxic effects of plant fiber. *The American Journal of Clinical Nutrition* 27:1395, 1974.

——— and Marshall, W. E. Protective effects of dietary fiber in rats fed toxic doses of sodium cyclamate and polyoxyethylene sorbitan monostearate (Tween 60). *Journal of Food Science,* March–April 1975.

Groen, J. J. Why bread in the diet lowers serum cholesterol. *Proceedings Nutrition Society* 32:159, 1973.

Heaton, K. W. Are we getting too much out of food? *Nutrition* 27:170, 1973.

——— and Pomare, E. W. Effect of bran on blood lipids and calcium. *The Lancet,* pp. 49–50, 1974.

Irving, D., and Drasar, B. S. Fibre and cancer of the colon. *British Journal of Cancer* 28:462, 1973.

James, W. P. T. Food and death-rates from diabetes. *The Lancet,* pp. 1201–1202, 1974.

——— and Cummings, J. H. Dietary fibre and energy regulation. *The Lancet,* pp. 61–62, 1974.

Jones, A. F., and Godding, E. W. *Management of Constipation.* Oxford, 1972.

Keys, A. Sucrose in the diet and coronary heart disease. *Atherosclerosis* 14:193, 1971.

Kirwan, W. O., et al. Action of different bran preparations on colonic function. *British Medical Journal* 2:187, 1974.

McConnell, A. A., et al. Physical characteristics of vegetable foodstuffs that could influence bowel function. *Journal of the Science of Food and Agriculture* 25:1457, 1974.

——— and Eastwood, M. A. A comparison of methods of measuring 'fibre' in vegetable material. *Journal of the Science of Food and Agriculture* 25:1451, 1974.

Painter, N. S. Pressures in the colon related to diverticular disease. *Proceedings Royal Society of Medicine* 63:144, 1970.

———. *Diverticular disease of the colon—a disease of Western civilization.* Disease-a-Month. Chicago: Year Book Medical Publishers, June 1970.

——— and Burkitt, D. P. Diverticular disease of the colon: a deficiency disease of Western civilization. *British Medical Journal* 2:450, 1971.

——— et al. Unprocessed bran in treatment of diverticular disease of the colon. *British Medical Journal* 1:137, 1972.

———. The high fibre diet in the treatment of diverticular disease of the colon. *Postgraduate Medical Journal* 50:629, 1974.

Pomare, E. W., and Heaton, K. W. Alteration of bile salt metabolism by dietary fibre. *British Medical Journal* 4:262, 1973.

Southgate, D. A. T. Fibre in nutrition. *Bibliotheca Nutritio et Dieta,* No. 22, p. 109, 1975.

———. Dietary Fibre. *Plant Foods for Man,* Autumn 1973.

Strasberg, S. M., and Fisher, M. M. Pathogenesis of human cholesterol cholelithiasis. *Canadian Medical Association Journal* 112:484, 1975.

Trowell, H. A case of coronary heart disease in an African. *East African Medical Journal* 33:393, 1956.

———. *Non-infective Disease in Africa.* London: Edward Arnold, 1960.

———. Ischemic heart disease and dietary fiber. *The American Journal of Clinical Nutrition* 25:926, 1972.

———. Crude fibre, dietary fibre and atherosclerosis. *Atherosclerosis* 16:138, 1972.

———. Guest editorial and general review: Dietary fibre and coronary heart disease. *European Journal of Clinical and Biological Research* 17:345, 1972.

———. Dietary fibre, ischaemic heart disease and diabetes mellitus. *Proceedings Nutrition Society* 32:151, 1973.

———. Fibre and obesity. *The Lancet,* p. 95, Jan. 19, 1974.

———. Definitions of fibre. *The Lancet,* p. 503, March 23, 1974.

———. Diabetes mellitus death-rates in England and Wales, 1920–70 and food supplies. *The Lancet,* p. 998, Oct. 26, 1974.

———. Dietary fibre, coronary heart disease and diabetes mellitus. *Plant Foods for Man,* Spring 1974.

Van Soest, P. J., and McQueen, R. W. The chemistry and estimation of fibre. *Proceedings Nutrition Society* 32:123, 1973.

Walker, A. R. P. The effect of recent changes of food habits on bowel motility. *South African Medical Journal,* p. 590, August 23, 1947.

———. Diet and atherosclerosis. *The Lancet,* p. 565, March 12, 1955.

———. Some aspects of nutritional research in South Africa. *Nutrition Reviews* 14:321, 1956.

———. Crude fibre, bowel motility, and pattern of diet. *South African Medical Journal* 35:114, 1961.

———. Bowel motility and colonic cancer. *British Medical Journal* 3:238, 1969.

———. Bowel transit times in Bantu populations. *British Medical Journal* 3:48, 1970.

———. Sugar intake and coronary heart disease. *Atherosclerosis* 14:137, 1971.

———. Diet, bowel motility, faeces composition and colonic cancer. *South African Medical Journal* 45:377, 1971.

——— et al. Appendicitis, fibre intake and bowel behavior in ethnic groups in South Africa. *Postgraduate Medical Journal* 49:243, 1973.

———. The bran hypothesis. *The Lancet,* p. 341, Aug. 10, 1974.

———. Request editorial: Dietary fibre and the pattern of diseases. *Annals of Internal Medicine* 80:663, 1974.

———. Editorial: The epidemiological emergence of ischemic arterial diseases. *American Heart Journal* 89:133, 1975.

Yudkin, J. *Pure white and deadly*. London: Davis-Poynter, 1972.

General Index

Recipe Index